**Psychosocial
Counseling
in General
Medical Practice**

Psychosocial Counseling in General Medical Practice

Allen Hodges
University of Colorado

Lexington Books
D.C. Heath and Company
Lexington, Massachusetts
Toronto

Library of Congress Cataloging in Publication Data

Hodges, Allen.
  Psychosocial counseling in general medical practice.

  1. Psychotherapy. 2. Counseling. 3. Physicians (General practice) I. Title.
[DNLM: 1. Counseling. 2. General practice. 3. Physician—Patient relations.
W89 H688p]
RC480.H56   616.8'914   76-40401
ISBN 0-669-01039-1

Copyright © 1977 by D.C. Heath and Company

Published simultaneously in Canada

Printed in the United States of America

International Standard Book Number: 0-669-01039-1

Library of Congress Catalog Card Number: 76-40401

Contents

List of Tables

Foreword

This book is the product of interaction between two perceptive health care practitioners, seeking more efficient and effective means of helping general medical patients with psychosocial dilemmas. Dr Hodges has brought together a methodology for gathering psychosocial data in an efficient but sensitive manner, incorporating such data into a record system that helps the practitioner identify the full range of patient problems and outlines a method of pragmatic intervention into the psychosocial problems. Extensive use is made of the Minnesota Multiphasic Personality Inventory (MMPI), drawing upon the vast body of data that has been collected on that instrument.

This effort makes an important contribution to the growing literature in the health field that has resulted from the introduction of Weed's Problem-Oriented System. During the past half decade there has been widespread adoption of the Problem-Oriented System (POS). Almost all medical students receive some training in the system. In the psychosocial field, mental health centers, academic departments of psychiatry, state and private hospitals as well as private practitioners have adopted POS.

This book demonstrates the extended use of POS as a bridge for the health care provider in order to identify and list psychosocial health care concerns/problems at a pragmatic or functional level of definition, integrating such problems into a more complete patient health protocol.

This process of recognition of psychosocial problems, and the development of a method for systematic display of progress in solution of these problems, together with their interaction with medical/physical problems of a patient, is a highly innovative contribution of this book.

Throughout the many case examples, Dr. Hodges has demonstrated the importance of including problem listings *at basic descriptive levels*. If a family practitioner is presented data from the patient suggesting marital difficulties, job dissatisfaction, difficulty with assertiveness, lack of sexual satisfaction, or lack of close friends, then these descriptions are included in the problem list. That the patient may have a depressive neurosis, or schizophrenia, or a passive-aggressive personality, is irrelevant for naming the patient's problems. Certainly a psychiatric diagnosis may be highly relevant when it comes to deciding *how* to intervene in these problems, but the problem itself remains, irrespective of diagnosis. The use of psychiatric nomenclature to attempt to describe or identify specific patient problems has come under attack from many quarters, and rightfully so. Standard psychiatric diagnoses do not function well in identifying or describing the multiple dilemmas or concerns which may need attention if the patient is to receive comprehensive health care. The emphasis of this book—encouraging the health care provider to focus upon pragmatic psychosocial problems expressed by the patient, rather than engaging in high level psychiatric diagnostic formulations—has an important message.

Psychosocial Counseling in General Medical Practice should serve as a useful complement to the continuing education of those primary care providers who wish to increase their skills in psychosocial problem identification and intervention. Whether the physician sees himself or herself as the primary intervener in patients' psychosocial problems or refers them, is relatively unimportant. The crucial step of *recognition* of psychosocial problems and their *interaction* with medical/physical problems, incorporated into a comprehensive health plan for that patient, appears essential for the conscientious health practitioner.

The pragmatic problem-solving approach utilized throughout this book represents a marked contrast to the eduction most physicians have received during their formal medical training. In medical schools the thrust of most formal eductional efforts concerning psychosocial care is focused on psychiatric diagnostic categories, and exposure to highly theoretical conceptualizations aimed at understanding the origins of patient difficulties. Very little effort is expended on the skills of problem identification at the pragmatic level; nor on systematic, eclectic problem-solving efforts for identified psychosocial problems. Some practitioners, heavily indoctrinated by their previous training, may label the model presented in this book as simplistic, incomplete, fragmented, or inappropriate. However, for those primary care physicians who wish to pursue the psychosocial difficulties presented by their patients in the same problem-solving mode that they use for medical/physical problems, the model contained here provides a useable and satisfying technique.

It is hoped that this book may contribute to filling a learning deficit in the skills of non-psychiatric physicians. It is further hoped that present and future medical training will focus more upon the skills of physician-patient interaction, which is at the core of Dr. Hodges' contribution in this volume.

Richard L. Grant, M.D.
Associate Professor of Psychiatry
University of Colorado Medical Center
Denver, Colorado

Acknowledgments

I wish to publicly express my appreciation to Stuart L. Smith, M.D., who as friend, mentor, and collaborator introduced me to the area of general medical practice and the potential which exists for physician-psychologist collaboration. Historically, two individuals who contributed to my development must be acknowledged. T. Ernest Newland, Ph.D., influenced me greatly as a student and set a model of eclecticism which I have tended to follow; and the late Nathaniel J. Berkwitz, M.D., Ph.D., broadened my understanding of mind-body interaction, stressing the humaneness and compassion which must be present in order to perform as a healer.

Gratitude is offered to my wife who patiently and willingly tolerated World War II, my returning to school to obtain three degrees under the G.I. Bill, and who has dedicated herself for 32 years to my well-being and the well-bing of our four daughters. This book is dedicated to her.

Special thanks are offered to Robert Chandler, M.D., Harry Hoewischer, Ph.D., and Jerry Garland, M.D., for their editorial comments and suggestions, and to Jo Ann Lorenz who typed the final manuscript.

**Psychosocial
Counseling in
General Medical
Practice**

1

Introduction

Throughout America today there is an observable trend for individuals seeking health care to select primary physicians for their entry into the health care system. Many speculations might be offered to explain this relatively recent turn of events. Some may argue that the prime reason is economic. Certainly the recognition by the total medical community of the critical need for a broadly trained general practitioner who perceives the patient as a totality rather than as an appendage to a particular organ system has done much to encourage this development. From the patient's viewpoint there appears to be a more basic and somewhat simpler explanation.

In our present troubled time, where distrust of almost all institutions is prevalent, where depersonalization and the fear of being "ripped off" are almost universal attitudes, there appears to be a positive countercurrent existing in the mood of people. The desire to establish a personalized relationship with a trusted and skilled advocate to aid the patient to better cope with the stresses and complexities of modern day living seems to be a more plausible reason for the increased reliance upon the primary physician. Some of the reasons verbalized by patients placing themselves under the care of such a physician are to aid the patient in understanding medical and psychological terms which he (the patient) hears spoken about his health care, to help the patient understand the complexities of the total health care system, and to give the patient a better grasp of his own problems in their proper perspective and priority. Such an expanded role for the primary physician in rendering comprehensive care to his patients, however, brings many additional professional headaches and responsibilities. One of the most immediate and perplexing of these is the intertwining of physical and emotional aspects of human behavior—in sickness or in health.

Since the beginning of written history, this problem has plagued mankind. Whether "mind" and "body" are separate, parallel, or of the same substance was a major concern of ancient philosophers and metaphysicians. It is, in the twentieth century, still of prime importance. There is a resurgence of pseudo-scientific "systems" to explain the mind-body dilemma through such outside forces as the position of the sun and the moon in our horoscope. According to

1

a 1975 Gallup Poll, some 20 million Americans, or approximately 10 percent of the adult population, believe astrology to be a partial answer to their moods and feelings of well-being. At the other end of the continuum, modern bio-chemists, neurophysiologists, and psychopharmocologists continue the scientific quest to discover linkages between the psyche and soma.

As the primary physician attempts to provide comprehensive care to his patients, the foremost problem that he will immediately encounter will be in his dealings with the patient's temperament, his attitudinal belief systems, his environmental stresses, his habits, and his style of life. Out of the present morass of personality theories, philosophical writings, and highly technical research findings, the primary physician will be forced to develop a sound theory of health and a practical and straightforward approach to the diagnosis and ame-lioration of emotional-behavioral aspects of his patient's health problems. Any approach adopted must be grounded upon sound medical and psychological practice. It must also be rational and acceptable to the patient.

The procedures, practices, and techniques reported derived from collabora-tion and the mutual efforts of a primary physician and a clinical psychologist. Over a three-year period of experimentation, trial and error, these approaches and techniques gradually evolved. To both collaborators, the experience of working with a colleague of a different professional orientation, the product of a different educational process, was gratifying and contributed to the growth of both. The end result has been the development of a theory and a rational strategy to deal with emotional-behavioral problems of selected general medical patients which includes aspects of both medical and psychological orientation.

The primary physician had served as a general practitioner in rural Colorado for 15 years before entering a general surgical residency and becoming Boarded as a General Surgeon. In his efforts to provide comprehensive health care to general medical patients, he had concluded that a problem-oriented approach to the practice of medicine made immediate sense. The frequency and persistence of emotional-behavioral problems occurring within the health protocols of his patients motivated the physician to seek alternatives to the present ones of re-ferring the patient to public or private mental health service providers. The surgical background of the physician, in addition to his role as primary health provider, will be evident in the contents of case history material.

The clinical psychologist had spent over 20 years in school psychological services and in psychiatric and mental health settings, and was actively seeking a new, more challenging setting for interacting with individuals experiencing emotional or behavioral difficulties. Of particular interest was the utilization of psychodiagnostic techniques with "normal" populations, the use of brief psycho-therapeutic counseling techniques, and primary prevention in mental health.

Through a mutual friend, who was aware of the physician's somatopsychic interests and the psychologist's psychosomatic interests, the two met. Both had been influenced by the earlier writings of Ward Darley.[1] In addition to com-

mon professional interests, the collaborators were also drawn together by the
tenor of the times—emphasis upon cost effectiveness in health care, Title XVIII
and XIX, PSROs, third party providers, the need for more innovative efforts in
comprehensive health care as opposed to the treatment of disease.

It may appear presumptuous that two individuals, without the resources of
a large medical foundation or a large number of clinical cases upon which to
draw, could contribute to the art and practice of comprehensive patient care.
This attitude, particularly on the part of practitioners who undertake the day-
to-day responsibilites of dealing with the patient as a person, should be reasses-
sed. It is doubtful that the provision of quality medical care will emerge solely
from the laboratory or in the computer room. Significant contributions in the
art of rendering primary health care will likely take place in the face-to-face
encounters between patient and practitioner.

Another point should be made concerning the collaborative undertakings
between professionals of differing orientations. In addition to the long range
aim of aiding the patient, there must exist certain "bridge concepts" that will
enable linkages to take place between different bodies of knowledge. The
problem-oriented medical approach provides one such link between physician
and psychologist. An objective and reliable personality classification system is
another bridge between the two collaborators to better understand each other
and to determine the patient's emotional makeup.

The problem-oriented approach to primary care is of such importance that
Chapters 2 and 3 are devoted exclusively to this procedure. The necessity for
an objective and reliable psychodiagnostic tool that is acceptable to general
medical patients without conveying negative anxiety-provoking reactions is
described in Chapter 4. The utilization of brief psychotherapeutic/counseling
procedures, requiring one to ten visits within the environment of the general
medical setting, is described in Chapter 5. The rediscovery of brief psychotherapeutic intervention developed in the 1940s is a particularly fruitful method of
dealing with the emotional/behavioral problems of general medical patients.

The evolution of "style of life" counseling/psychotherapy rendered by
physician, psychologist, or both, is discussed in depth in Chapter 6. In many
instances, individuals are encountered in general medical settings who have no
diagnosable organic disease, nor suffer any incapacitating emotional disorder,
yet the patient's lifestyle strongly suggests that help is needed to develop alternatives, to anticipate and prepare for future roles, or to reassess life priorities if
more serious health problems are to be prevented.

Chapters 7 through 10 deal with common emotional/behavioral problems
of general medical patients. Depression and grief, interpersonal problems, psychoneurosis, and borderline psychotic states are the topics for separate chapters.
Chapter 11 again addresses the mind-body question, and suggests areas for
future collaboration between physician and psychologist. In each chapter, case
histories are used to emphasize and stress salient points.

Summary

In attempting to sum up the major aim of this undertaking, it is hoped that the chapters that follow will enable the primary care physician and the psychologist to obtain a better concept of exploring and dealing with the emotional and behavioral aspects of primary medical patients. The author also hopes that collaborative efforts between physician and psychologist will be further stimulated as we strive toward better definitions of primary and comprehensive care.

It would appear from most of the current proposals being debated in Congress and by the man on the street that "quality of care" is primarily a political and organizational problem, which can be solved by "programming" delivery of services in a cost efficient manner. It may seem extremely old-fashioned, but there is evidence to support the belief that there are greater possibilities in existence to upgrade the quality of care by improving the primary physician's skill in the early detection and prevention of debilitating disease.

Whether the physician is practicing in a health maintenance organization, a large metropolitan city, or an isolated rural area, the quality of medical care is highly dependent upon the physician's interpersonal skills and competencies in dealing with the patient as a total person. One of the obvious medical enigmas is the fact that unless the patient enters willingly into the diagnostic treatment and preventive processes, quality of care then becomes an empty slogan. Clearly, one of the major requirements for upgrading the quality of primary medical care is for the health delivery system to become more competent in its dealings with the human aspects of the patient. It is within this specific area that a meshing of medicine and psychology will likely occur within the next decade. Perhaps at this basic and functional level, more learning can take place concerning the nature of man than from philosophical speculation.

References

1. See Darley, Ward, and Barnacle, C.H. Association of the Internist and Psychiatrist in Private Practice. *American Journal of Medical Science*, 201(1941): 86–92. See also Darley, Ward. American Medicine and its Responsibility. *Rocky Mountain Medical Journal*, 43(1945):464–65; The Place and Training of the General Practitioner. *California Medicine*, 70(1949):265–268; Medical Education, Specialty Practice, and The Family Doctor. *Rocky Mountain Medical Journal*, 49(1952):1–6; We Need a New Specialty: Family Practice. *New Medica Materia*, March 1962, p. 29; Relationship of Psychiatry to Problems of Medical Care. *Diseases of The Nervous System*, VIII(1967):2–4; Allied Health Personnel and Their Employment in the Improvement of Medical Care. *New England Journal of Medicine*, 281(1969):443–45.

2

Problem-oriented Medicine— Theory and Practice

The Problem Oriented Medical Information System developed by Lawrence L. Weed[1] is an ideal method with which to begin the study of the interaction of physical, emotional, and behavioral factors in general medical patients. Weed's POMIS is based upon the systematic collection of pertinent data from which inferences and treatment plans are made. The logic and clarity of POMIS in clinical practice is obvious. Less obvious, but perhaps more important in the long run, is the structure POMIS provides for action-oriented research, interprofessional collaboration, and long range evaluation. Weed's POMIS contains four major sections:

1. the routine collection of meaningful data concerning the patient;
2. the formulation of a problem list, with the rank ordering of health problems from most severe to less severe;
3. the development of treatment plans for each of the health problems contained in the patient's problem list; and
4. followup of changes over time within each health problem area, based upon patient reports, laboratory findings, and observed medical changes.

Guilford[2] has proposed that five basic processes, separately or in combination, are involved in all forms of intellectual activity, including problem solving. It is interesting to assess Weed's contribution to the practice of comprehensive health care from the viewpoint of Guilford's five intellectual processes.

Guildford's first intellectual operation is labeled *Cognitive Thinking.* In its simplest form, cognitive skill or intellectual capacity is the ability to detect relationships and to infer meaning from such observations. "Creativity" and "perceptiveness" are two synonyms that convey aspects of cognition. The professions of the healing sciences offer many opportunities for cognitive skills. Unless observations are strictly intuitive in nature, however, some method is essential that will allow standardization of observations and the testing of relationships. In the history of the development of any science, the systematic recording of observable data formed the basis upon which later scientific developments occur. Weed's POMIS provides such a format, allowing the

5

physician to record meaningful data and to systematically ask cognitive relationship types of questions.

Memory is Guilford's second intellectual operation. Memory, of course, depends upon prior experience, and the working through of problems at an earlier time. As one views clinical training in retrospect, the opportunity to learn first hand through clinical experiences under supervision was ultimately aimed at providing meaningful experiences that could be stored in one's "memory bank" for future problem-solving situations. To overly rely upon memory, even with one patient and his complex of symptoms, is extremely risky in the healing professions. Weed's POMIS augments clinical memory by routinely requiring the physician to record basic information about the patient and his specific health problem rather than committing such details to memory.

A third intellectual operation proposed by Guilford is termed *Divergent Thinking*. In its simplest form, it might be thought of as "many ways to skin a cat" intelligence. As an example, take Laser's highly cognitive discovery of the Laser Beam, produced by routing light rays through a ruby. The potential applications of the use of the Laser Beam represents a different intellectual process than the highly cognitive and creative ability required to conceive it. Within the development of the medicine, there are many examples of divergent thinking. Recognition that neural impulses follow principles of electricity developed in physics, and the transferring of engineering principles to the design of an artificial heart or in orthopedic restructuring, are but two examples. Weed's POMIS is itself an example of divergent thinking, in which he has "transferred" techniques that have evolved out of systems analysis and "management by objectives" and applied such principles to the practice of medicine. In the process, Weed's POMIS provides a framework whereby medical practitioners may obtain a broader view of the interrelationships and changes that may occur in seemingly unrelated health problem areas as a result of intervention in one specific health problem.

A fourth intellectual process or problem-solving method has been designated as *Convergent Thinking*. While divergent solutions have many "right" answers, convergent solutions have only one. The process of differential diagnosis, observation of specific symptoms, and organizing such symptoms into a hypothesis of a specific diagnosis is the sine qua non of convergent thinking. It must be remembered however, that such a convergent reasoning process assumes that there *is* a single cause lying at the root of the many symptoms. Perhaps the germ theory of disease causality enhanced during the early 1900s has overstressed this intellectual process in medicine. As we shall see in Chapter 3, the major health problems of the 1970s—cancer, heart, alcoholism—appear to be the result of *multiple* causes. Still, the convergent reasoning process is an essential problem-solving method of the physician, and Weed's POMIS provides a systematic method wherein differential diagnoses can occur.

The final intellectual process proposed by Guilford is *Evaluation*. A problem may be tackled in cognitive, memory, convergent, or divergent style, but the ultimate conclusion as to the adequacy of the problem solving rests with evaluative skills. Medicine has been criticized for not foreseeing long range implications of practices and procedures aimed at producing short range remissions of specific illnesses. The crisis intervention nature of the physician's efforts to cope with patient emergencies is largely responsible for this criticism. Weed's POMIS, collecting basic medical data on each patient and longitudinally following the patient's progress within specified health areas over time, can do much to strengthen the evaluative process in patient care.

Viewing POMIS as an umbrella system that provides the framework within which all forms of problem-solving approaches can be utilized in the care and treatment of patients emphasizes the magnitude of Weed's contribution to medical practice. Adopted by the primary physician, POMIS could be the foundation upon which increased research efforts could be undertaken related to patient care.

But what about the patient? What does a problem-oriented approach mean to him or her? It is all well and good that a technique is invaluable to the practitioner, but if the patient feels that the technique is too time-consuming, too expensive, or too intimate or threatening in terms of personal information required, the utility of such a technique is limited. The experiences reported in this book suggest that even in exploring the most sensitive areas of the patients' life problems, particularly in Phases Two and Three of POMIS, most patients express gratitude to the physician who takes the time to obtain the patients' views and judgments. The importance of *joint* physician-patient rankings in POMIS is perhaps a key psychological process within the total problem-oriented system.

Formulation of a Health Problem Protocol

Almost 90 percent of patients appearing in the primary physician's office for the first time verbalize some specific complaint as the reason for seeking medical care. Reasons for seeking medical attention may range from "rectal bleeding" to such general complaints as "sleeping poorly," "tension," or "weight loss or gain." The physician, after listening to the patient's description of the specific health complaint, proceeds to undertake a physical history and examination of the patient, conducting the necessary laboratory and physical tests that his judgment dictates to collect the necessary medical information demanded in constructing the routine and unique data base required for that patient. (A rich source of meaningful medical-psychological research is the presenting complaints of patients seeking primary physician care. If the hypothesis is correct that there is a strong underlying need for many prospective patients to establish a relationship with a health care provider who will serve as his advocate and advisor, then the "presenting complaint" could possibly provide an indicator of those patients who perceive the primary physician as a crisis interviewer [disease treater] as opposed to those who are seeking a broader role for the primary physician as a health advocate.)

Phase Two of POMIS, from a psychological viewpoint, is perhaps the most critical in the ultimate outcome of the entire process. The primary physician, integrating the physical, laboratory, and diagnostic findings, interprets to the patient the results and the physician's hypotheses as to the patient's overall health status and a breakdown of the specific health problems that the physician's findings indicate.

If the process stops at this point, with the all-knowing physician developing a health priority list *for* the patient, then the primary physician has set the boundaries as to what aspects of the patient's life *he* (the physician) is interested in, what *he* (the physician) feels competent to deal with, and what *he* (the physician as "expert") feels are the primary health problems of the patient.

If one views the formulation of a health problem protocol as a *joint* venture between the primary physician and the patient, this approach alone is perhaps the pivotal point as to whether the physician is practicing disease-oriented medicine or striving to offer comprehensive health care. If the patient is perceived as a full partner in his or her present and future health care, then the patient must also contribute to the final development of a listing of health problems. As a partner in formulating a listing of health problems, the patient also must perceive that treatment or amelioration of identified health problems is also a joint responsibility, with the physician acting as counselor-teacher-evaluator and the patient assuming responsibility for the day-to-day execution of treatment plans.

If this premise is accepted—*that the patient must be a full partner in the formulation and plans for amelioration of his own health problems*—then many vistas become open to the primary physician. Accepting the fact that the patient is the ultimate authority as to *his* sources of pain, *his* discomforts, *his* attitudes of well-being and feelings of health, then the patient's full participation in the ordering of health problems begins to approximate health care as opposed to disease or disease prevention practice.

If the problem listing is a mutual product of patient and primary physician then the physician will immediately observe what might be termed "an apples and oranges phenomenon." A patient may rank order a seemingly "insignificant" problem such as "problems in communicating with wife" much higher in priority than an apparent life-threatening health condition. This is perhaps a truism, but pain and discomfort are not exclusively biological phenomena. The pain and discomfort of a family interpersonal conflict upon a middle-aged, anxious mother may far exceed the physical discomforts of a medically diagnosed life-threatening health problem.

Taking the patient into the problem formulation process as a full partner does not imply that the primary physician does not attempt to change and reorder the patient's perception of his health priorities. On the contrary, the physician as a tutor and educator utilizes all of his interpersonal and professional skills in attempting to help his patient obtain a broader, more realistic integration of health problems. As clinical case histories will indicate, this process may occur over weeks, months, years, or perhaps never.

Summary

POMIS and its potential scientific contribution to primary medical care has been strongly stressed. Psychologically, taking the patient as a full partner into the problem formulation process is equally important. When a mutually developed health problem listing is completed, the primary physician has before him a gamut of comprehensive health/emotional/social/behavioral problems that are unique to the patient. With the patient participating as full partner, the stage is then set for the formulation of patient-physician treatment plans.

The primary physician contributes his knowledge in discerning those problems amenable to the medical health therapies. *The primary physician, if he is to render comprehensive care, must accept such emotional/behavioral health problems upon which the patient places high priority and for which he asks eradication or relief, as sources of pain and discomfort and must aid the patient in formulating treatment plans.*

If emotional/behavioral problems are rejected as legitimate concerns of the primary physician, then the patient will seek help for such problems elsewhere. In the process, he will quickly learn where the physician's interests really lie and will return to the physician only in physical crisis situations. Any preventive suggestions or health-nurturing advice by such a medically oriented primary physician will likely be interpreted by the patient as well-meaning advice but far removed from the patient's "real" problems.

Procedures

Using the rational approach described through the use of POMIS, the primary physician associated with this project encouraged the patient to include emotional/behavioral problems within his health problem listing. In working with the patient to develop treatment plans for each health problem identified, the primary physician treated such emotional/behavioral health problems in exactly the same manner as conventional physical problems. If the patient indicated a desire for help, the primary physician scheduled an appointment for the patient to confer with the clinical psychologist located within the same general office setting. Prior to the first interview with the patient, the psychologist had the patient complete the MMPI (Minnesota Multiphasic Personality Inventory) in the general medical office. The MMPI was scored and the results entered into the patient's general medical file. Prior to the first patient-psychologist interview, the complete case file was reviewed by the psychologist and discussed with the primary physician. This was the underpinning for psychosocial counseling interactions with each patient.

References

1. Weed, Lawrence C. *Medical Records, Medical Education, and Patient Care*. Cleveland: Case Western Reserve University Press, 1969.

2. Guilford, J.P. Three Faces of Intellect. *American Psychologist* 14(1959): 469–79; also Guilford, J.P. Intelligence: 1965 Model. *American Psychologist* 21 (1966):20–26.

3

Behavioral/Emotional Components in General Practice

In June 1975, the U.S. Public Health Service published "Forward Planning for Health." Contrasts between 1900 and the present as to the leading causes of death illustrate how medical problems have changed during that period. Pneumonia, influenza, and tuberculosis, the early killers, have now been replaced by diseases of the heart and malignant neoplasms. Today tuberculosis ranks twenty-first as the cause of death.

Most of today's health problems are caused by a variety of factors not susceptible to medical solutions or to direct intervention by the health practitioner: we have no vaccine to prevent cancer or to cure alcoholism. This poses a dilemma for health professionals in defining a proper role for themselves in the prevention of disease and a practical problem for those concerned with setting the boundaries of health planning. For planning purposes, it is not realistic to view smoking primarily as a medical problem. It is a major social, economic, cultural and psychological phenomenon that has profound health implications.[1]

The report goes further into the analysis of deaths and injuries produced by automobile accidents, alcoholism, inadequate or excessive food consumption, environmental pollution, and physical inactivity. The conclusions drawn are essentially the same for smoking. The "causes" of these health problems are rooted in social, economic, cultural, and psychological areas. The report further points out that as rising unemployment and economic recession continues, one can, with statistical confidence, predict increases in child abuse, crime, suicide, and homicide. Within the population below 20 years of age, the tremendous increases in venereal disease, deaths by violence, drug abuse, all ultimately resulting in medical problems, have their origins in cultural and social areas that then become incorporated into the psychological and behavioral makeup of the individual. In addition to these recent cultural phenomena, the age-old problems of marital conflict, interfamily crises, grief, sex dysfunctions, work maladjustment, and adjustments to aging continue to produce psychic pain and tension, probably lowering resistance to disease.

As a problem-oriented approach is taken to general medical populations, and particularly where patient and physician jointly attempt to rank order health

11

and medical problems, a more objective and a more realistic appraisal of emotional/behavioral components can be undertaken. To eliminate these behavioral/emotional factors from medical concern is to constrict the primary physician to being a treater of physical diseases and abrogates the tremendous impact that the patient-physician relationship can produce in the prevention of disease and illness. To attempt to categorize patient complaints in an "either-or" manner, either physical or emotional, is to accept a rather simplistic view of human behavior. The blatant statement that "seventy percent of all complaints of patients in a general medical setting are emotional in origin" is a rather destructive generalization. It implies a dichotomy between feelings and pain, illness and attitudes, stress and physiologic reaction, all of which weaken the practice of preventive medicine. More and more general medical patients, having read the latest article in some weekly exposé newspaper or magazine article on psychosomatic diseases, preface the discussion with a sheepish introduction such as, "This is probably nothing more than nerves, but I feel . . . !" As the mind-body dichotomy is perpetuated through the popular media, one wonders how much valuable clinical data is being suppressed by patients when they are encouraged to discuss health and health-related concerns and fears.

Statistically, if one includes smoking, dietary habits, safety attitudes, and alcohol and drug misuse as legitimate concerns of the general medical/family practitioner, then the probabilities are less than one in 56 that a patient in a general setting is totally free of these potential health hazards. If the ongoing problems of divorce and marital disharmony, job stress, and sex dysfunction are added to this problem listing, then the probabilities jump to one in 3,216 of a patient being completely free of any of the potential stresses that these conditions provide!

A review of a sample of general medical records confirms this observation, and suggests that a mere elaboration of emotional/behavioral concerns listed as problems among general medical patients will add little to understanding the interplay between emotional/behavioral factors and health/disease. Instead, selected case records provide a better method for illustrating this interaction.

The Case of Tim

This 46-year-old married Caucasian male first sought medical attention for internal and external hemorrhoids. He had previously received injections for his condition, which had worsened in the past three months. He is currently employed in the news department of a large metropolitan radio station. Stresses on the job have increased during the past six months. Severe disagreements exist between the patient, who desires to reliably verify all news intems prior to broadcast, and the radio station's manager, who desires to be first on the air with the news. The patient's wife does not want to move to a different part of the country, and so the patient feels considerable pressure to continue his present job, despite the stresses. Since the patient devotes most of his waking hours to work, there is no time for hobbies or other non-job-related outlets. The patient has 20 separate radio receivers in his living room so that he can monitor police and radio channels as well as competitor radio stations.

A physical examination revealed an essentially healthy individual. Barium enema and Bilirubin/amylase revealed no abnormalities.

With the participation of the patient, the following problems were developed in a rank order, from most important to least important:

1. Hemorrhoids
2. Periodic pain from herniated disc from ski injury
3. Stress on the job
4. Chronic anxiety and sleeplessness

The patient decided that he would enter the hospital and have the hemorrhoids surgically treated. This was accomplished two weeks after the patient's first outpatient visit. The surgeon's report is as follows:

This patient had huge masses of prolapsing internal and external hemorrhoids and had previously had injection treatment. The large donut of anal tissue remained. A sigmoidoscopy was done, the entire length of the scope inserted and no mucosal abnormalities demonstrated. The prostate was normal. Seminal vesical was not palpable. The dorsal midline sphineterotomy was done. Stick ties were placed laterally and anteriorly and a Parks-type circumferential submucosal hemorrhoidectomy was performed removing both internal and external hemorroids and a large amount of tissue. Bleeding was controlled with electrocautery. A few sutures were used to align the mucosa inside the dentate line. The estimated blood loss was 200 to 250 ccs. Xylocaine viscus apparatus was put in place. A pressure dressing was applied. The patient returned to the recovery room in good condition.

With the usual complaints of pain of excretion, patient's stay in the hospital was uneventful and he was released five days after surgery. A week following hospital discharge, the patient was seen for postoperative checkup. He still complained of some pain after bowel movement but healing appeared well advanced and a monthly followup visit was scheduled. Two days after this visit, the patient awakened in the night extremely apprehensive and sweating profusely. His wife, who suspected a heart attack, called an ambulance, and he was rushed to the emergency room. Examination revealed no cardiac problems, and hyperventilation and anxiety appeared as the causal factors. With reassurance by the attending medical personnel, his attack abated and he was released two hours later. This patient continued to suffer anxiety attacks for the next six months, at periodic intervals, and was fired from the news department of the radio station and became quite depressed. After three months of seeking another position and with encouragement and therapy from his physician and psychologist, the patient obtained a better paying job in the East. In the year since his move, he has telephoned twice to report that he is succeeding in his current job and that while he still feels tinges of the panic and anxiety that caused hyperventilation, he is able to control the severity of the anxiety without medication.

Without probing the theoretical psychic causes of Tim's emotional problems, his case represents the changing importance of emotional/behavioral factors to his medical well-being. A month prior to his firing from his job, the job stresses, while recognized, were far below his physical concerns of hemorrhoids and pain from an old back injury. With the added stress of being fired from his job, this exacerbated the pent-up affect that had been building for some time, shifting the priorities of his concern from a prime physical problem to a foremost emotional/behavioral problem. This shifting of importance of patients' emotional complaints and physical health concerns in a commonly observed process and one that the practitioner must be aware of and follow over periods of time.

The Case of Jan

Jan is a 42-year-old housewife who has worked 20 to 25 hours per week outside the home for the past four years. She has four children ranging in ages from 12 to 23. Her husband, age 50, is physically well and has many outdoor hobbies including hunting and fishing. The patient has no hobbies. Previous surgery includes hysterectomy at age 41, and an appendectomy 10 years earlier. No family history of breast cancer, rheumatic fever, or diabetes. The reason for seeking medical care is Problem No. 1.

Problem No. 1. Epigastric pain associated with a lump, subcostal midline, brought on with or without food.
Problem No. 2. Rectal fullness due to excessive mucous, present for the past three years.
Problem No. 3. Daily anxiety with marked hyperactivity, with feeling of "can't settle down" (constriction around area of the thyroid appears to accompany such feelings).
Problem No. 4. Surgical menopause, sensations of "hot flashes," even with injections of estrogen.

G.I. series revealed no abnormalities, only the notation that "patient's stomach is quite large, and the patient had lost 30 pounds through dieting during past twelve months."

During the next three months, problems 1 and 2 were treated medically and through diet. In bi-weekly visits on an outpatient basis, it was observed that as the patient's physical problems 1 and 2 began to abate, problem 3, anxiety and hyperactivity, appeared to increase. This observation led to a discussion with the patient of the possibility of interaction between problems 1, 2, and 3, and the need to explore problem 3 in more depth. This was accepted by the patient readily with the statement, "I've known for a long time that my feelings were tied into those physical pains, but didn't want to say it for fear that I'd be called 'Nuts'." Brief counseling was initiated, and problem 3 was explored in more depth. The patient in describing herself said, "Since I can remember I get all 'bottled up' and let resentments build up until they become so strong, I feel like I'm going to explode." In the course of personality assessment, it was felt that all four of Jan's problems were so intertwined and interrelated as to be inseparable, physically and emotionally. Psychotherapy, medication including a mood elevator, estrogen therapy, dietary changes, and reassessment of her part-time job were instituted, and improvement was obtained in a period of six weeks. It became apparent that much of Jan's anxiety and depression centered around her changing role as a mother and wife, and a lack of emotional communication with her husband, and that considerable apprehension existed as to her future happiness when her 10-year-old child became an adult and left home for good. The "empty nest" syndrome is well recognized as an extreme stress to mothers of large families. While Jane is not "cured," her problem balance appears to be in check, and hopefully if this homeostatic balance is again upset (as it is likely to be), she will return for further treatment and support.

The Case of Dora

This 47-year-old housewife and former elementary school teacher sought medical help because of arthritic pain in the neck, right arm, and fingers; feelings of depression and hopelessness; and menopausal reactions following vaginal hysterectomy three years ago. She is happily married to a school principal and has two living children, a girl 12 years of age and a boy aged 20. A third son, age 18 at the time of his death, was killed in an automobile accident five years previously. Physical examination and laboratory findings of the patient discovered no abnormalities. An arthritis profile revealed a positive reaction to rheumatoid factors. X-ray revealed normal chest and cervical spine readings. Slight osteoarthritis of the thoracic spine was revealed.

After compiling the physical examination results, including X-rays and laboratory test, the patient and physician attempted to assess and rank order the patient's concerns. The following problem list was jointly developed:

Problem No. 1. Depression and psychic pain over loss of son five years previously
Problem No. 2. Menopausal symptoms

Problem No. 3. Pain associated with arthritis in neck, right arm, and hand
Problem No. 4. Smoking and recurrent bronchitis
Problem No. 5. Heartburn experienced daily for the past ten years
Problem No. 6. Fear of cancer occurrence because of family history

In discussing Problem No. 1, the patient broke into tears at the recall of her son's death. She stated that neither she nor her husband could get over this loss. To the primary phycian, it appeared that Dora had not worked through her grief reaction to the accidental death of her son. This loss, which occurred five years ago, clouds her total health problem profile. In an effort to "get away from old memories" in the home in which the family had resided for the past 20 years, the patient and her husband bought a smaller older home. In the process of painting the interior of the newer residence, the patient overextended herself and attributes Problem No. 3 to this effort. Her smoking and recurrent bronchitis have been much more accentuated since her son's fatal accident.

Therapeutic procedures were taken to control Problem No. 2. When asked if she wished help concerning Problem No. 1, the patient declined counseling/therapy at that time although she completed psychodiagnostic procedures. In subsequent followup 18 months later, the patient appears to have her grief reactions and depression more under control and appears to be coping with her chronic medical problems. The mere process of the primary physician working jointly with Dora to evaluate the effects of her prolonged grief reaction upon her physical and emotional well-being appeared sufficient to help her regain an adequate state of health.

Summary

The three modified case histories were selected to illustrate varying physical/emotional interactions. In Tim, emotional problems lying dormant and for the most part under control suddenly emerge as a primary problem evoked by environmental stresses. At the time of seeking medical attention for his hemorrhoid problem and particularly in his post operative recovery phase, *both* the emotional/behavioral and the physical aspects of his pain had to be treated. The emotional problem has since receded and is now a problem of second and third magnitude. It remains, however, in his personality/biological makeup and subsequent physical difficulties and their treatment must take this emotional/behavioral component into account.

With Jan, it would appear that the emotional/behavioral aspects of her sources of pain are so intertwined with her physical and biological functioning that they must be treated jointly for either a physical or an emotional complaint.

In Dora, the external stress of the death of her 18-year-old son was such as to totally disrupt her physical and biological functioning. With time and compassionate understanding, the disruption of life from this emotional area appears to be receding, and she is beginning to experience joy and happiness. The emotional "scar" that the death of her son produced will *always* be there, and will likely be an ever-present factor in her physical and emotional well-being.

The role and importance of environmental stress and its concomitant effects upon the emotions, feelings, and physiology of people were major theoretical contributions of Adolph Meyer[2]. In 1967, Holmes and Rahe at the University of Washington School of Medicine devised a weighting system whereby stresses during the past 12 months could be assigned numerical weights[3]. Ranging from most stressful "death of a spouse" at 100 points, to "pregnancy" at 40 points, down to such minor stresses as "changing of sleeping habits" at 16 ponts and "minor violation of the law" at 11 points, Dr. Holmes and his colleagues have demonstrated the relationship between occurrence of serious illnesses (both physical and mental) and elevated scores on the social readjustment rating scale. As an adjunct to patient intake information, this rating scale can be readily obtained from the patient in a 15-minute self-administered format. Instruments such as this hold great promise in aiding the primary practitioner in obtaining a true feel for the patient, the stresses under which the patient operates, and potential sources of emotional pain.

References

1. *Forward Planning for Health.* U.S. Public Health Service, Deparment of Health, Education, and Welfare, June 1975, p. 97.

2. Meyer, A. A Psychobiologic Approach. *Journal of Mental Science* 79 (1933):435.

3. Holmes, T.H., and Rahe, R.H. The Social Readjustment Rating Scale. *Journal of Psychosomatic Research* 11(1967):213.

4

Integrating Psychodiagnosis into Problem-oriented Medicine

The lack of a commonly understood vocabulary and common orientation between the two disciplines concerning the emotional makeup and personality status of an individual has greatly handicapped effective interprofessional relatonships between psychologists and physicians. Perhaps more importantly, a lack of mutually understood concepts severely hampers the development of research from which improvements of the services to individual patients could evolve.

In a general office waiting room, either by a brief interview or by observation, certain behavioral manifestations of the patient's current emotional status can be easily ascertained. A simple rating scale can be devised to assess behavior in the office. Using a 5 point rating scale with 0 as a midpoint, +1, +2 to indicate the hyper range, and –1, –2 indicative of hypo activity, observations concerning the patient's tension level, mood, cooperativeness, and verbal responsiveness can be recorded. One must constantly keep in mind that such observed behavior may be situationally produced by the visit to the physician's office and may not be typical of the patient's behavior in other situations. For the purposes of substantiating such situational clinical observations and for the gathering of potential research data, it is necessary to have a standardized method by which personality and emotional assessment of a patient can be translated and communicated. Methods that depend upon subjective observations, interviews, or the use of constructs not understood by both communicator and hearer introduce inconsistencies or unreliability into the diagnostic process. Since validity, or accuracy in prediction, of *any* diagnostic process is dependent upon the reliability of the method, the use of a quantifiable and objective instrument is the first step in "proving" or "disproving" validity. This consistency problem is a critical one for personality assessors.

Beginning with the commonly observed phenomena that individuals behave differently in different situations, and therefore show different personality facets to their physician, their bartender, or their children, makes one hesitant to unequivocally select one of these situational "personalities" as genotypic. By common sense observation of ourselves and others, time, external factors, and stress *do* produce temporary and sometimes permanent personality changes.

19

"Personality," however, cannot be viewed as a changeable will-of-the-wisp phenomena or else there is no long range reason for even attempting to measure it. Neither can it be viewed as a rigid "cast iron" characteristic, impervious to change. The key concept that helps one out of this dilemma is what tests and measurement specialists refer to as "reliability."

Attention and effort varies from moment to moment. Over longer periods of time—weeks, months, years—changes occur on any test score in any area as a result of physical growth or decline, learning, changes in health status, or personality changes. Any technique, whether a patient-completed medical history sheet or a personality inventory, is subject to these change factors; hence the introduction of "inconsistencies" into the test-retest results. By the use of statistical procedures, the reliability of the test results over periods of time can be calculated.

The 1976 trial of Patty Hearst and the disparate conclusions of the court-appointed psychiatrists and psychologists as to her emotional status introduce another reliability concern. With only idiosyncratic experiences and unique theoretical orientations as a guide, each examiner, following observations of Patty Hearst, arrived at varying conclusions as to her ability to stand trial and her mental status. Another essential of the concept of reliability is *that the procedure be so standardized as to eliminate the idiosyncratic bias of the observer.*

If psychodiagnostic procedures are to add anything to the better understanding of the patient's physical, emotional, and behavioral makeup, the *process* by which such observations are obtained must be standardized. The *reliability* of the instrument or procedure must be demonstrated, keeping in mind that "personality" is a fluid concept. The *findings* or results of such procedures must be presented in such a manner as to preclude error in communication. Finally, the process must be *replicable* by different examiners with consistent results or with the same patient over periods of time so that individual changes can be tracked.

The Minnesota Multiphasic Personality Inventory

The Minnesota Multiphasic Personality Inventory (MMPI), developed in 1940 by Starke R. Hathaway, a clinical psychologist, and J. Charnley McKinley, a neurologist, is the instrument of choice in initial efforts to introduce psychodiagnostic procedures into a general medical setting[1]. Since its initial publication, the MMPI has been tried and proven in a variety of psychiatric, medical, business, and educational settings. The research on the utility, reliability, and validity of the MMPI constitutes a large block of effort currently expended in personality measurement and personality theory. Over 200 separate scales have been developed in addition to the nine original scales. Computerized scoring and interpretation is provided by several large companies[2]. Early in its history, the potential of this instrument in general medical settings was recognized[3].

Derivation of the MMPI

In 1940 Hathaway and McKinley compiled a listing of previously included items on personality questionnaires and personality inventories. The Woodworth Personal Data Sheet[4], the first personality measure, was utilized in World War I. The Bell Adjustment Inventory[5] and the Bernreuter Personality Test[6] were forerunners of the MMPI whose items were included in Hathaway and McKinley's item pool. Until the development of the MMPI, such "personality" inventories as the Bell, Woodworth, and Bernreuter efforts were constructed on an a priori basis. Since certain symptoms were associated with certain psychiatric diagnostic categories, an "inventory" of the patient's symptoms could be obtained and these reported symptoms of the patient could be compared to the known symptom complexes of hypochondrical patients, manic patients, etc. The test taker's ability to answer falsely or the ability of the patient to see the social/psychiatric implications of answering "true" to a question as "Do you wet the bed frequently?" was also evident.

To validate the a priori assumptions of previous personality inventories, the MMPI authors took a pragmatic approach. First, they selected criterion groups, comprised of over 800 patients suffering from clearly diagnosed (in the common opinion of a group of both psychologists and psychiatrists) psychiatric cases within the University of Minnesota Hospital. This vast pool of personality items were then administered to each individual suffering from a clearly diagnosed psychiatric illness. An item-by-item analysis was then performed to select those items that *statistically* differentiated hypochondrical patients from all other psychiatric categories. A normal sample of 724 subjects selected from visitors to the University of Minnesota Hospitals was also included in the analysis as a control. A total of 550 items, each item statistically differentiating certain diagnostic categories, comprised the final contents of the MMPI. In the course of this standarization process, surprises occurred. Items which on an a priori basis should be related to certain diagnostic categories, did not prove to be related. Also, seemingly innocuous items appeared to have discriminative power in differentiating different psychiatric conditions from normals. A false response to the question "I enjoy detective or mystery stories" is found to be statistically related to a diagnosis of Psychoneurosis, Conversion Hysteria rather than to other diagnostic categories. By developing 30 to 75 items from within the 550 total item pool that show significant statistical relationships with a criterion diagnostic category, a clinical scale was derived. Nine original scales were thus developed. The 550 items contain 26 categories of items that have been classified as to content and are displayed in Table 4–1.

This discussion of the derivation of the MMPI is to acquaint the reader with the painstaking efforts that have gone into the standardization and validation of the MMPI.

The MMPI Scales

The first form of the MMPI consisted of items printed on separate cards which the patient sorted into "true," "false," or "cannot say" categories. Today the booklet form with answer sheet is most utilized because of its speed in scoring.

Table 4–1
An Arbitrary Classification of MMPI Items by Content

Category	Content Area	Number of Items
1	General health	9
2	General neurologic symptoms	19
3	Cranial nerves	11
4	Motility and coordination	6
5	Sensibility	5
6	Vasomotor, trophic, speech secretory problems	10
7	Cardiorespiratory system	5
8	Gastrointestinal system	11
9	Genitourinary system	5
10	Habits	19
11	Family and marital relations	26
12	Occupational problems	18
13	Educational problems	12
14	Sexual attitudes	16
15	Religious attitudes	19
16	Political attitudes—law and order	46
17	Social attitudes	72
18	Affect, depressive	32
19	Affect, manic	24
20	Obsessive and compulsive states	15
21	Delusions, hallucinations, illusions, ideas of reference	31
22	Phobias	29
23	Sadistic, masochistic trends	7
24	Morale	33
25	Items primarily related to masculinity-femininity	55
26	Items to indicate whether the individual is trying to place himself in an improbable acceptable light	15

Source: Dahlstrom, W. Grant, George Schlager Welsh and Leona E. Dahlstrom, *An MMPI Handbook: Vol. I Clinical Interpretation. A Revised Edition.* Minneapolis, Minn.: University of Minnesota Press, 1972, p. 5. © 1972 by the University of Minnesota. Published by the Psychological Corporation. Reprinted by permission.

Computerized answer sheets have been developed and several companies will score and provide a computerized interpretation of the MMPI for a nominal fee.

The Four Validity Scales. The scales ?, L, F, and K represent efforts to estimate the test-taking attitudes of the test takers. The symbol ? merely stands for the number of test items left unanswered by the respondent. By not responding "true" or "false" to a particular item, the patient may fit in one of three categories: he may not understand the question, he may have no real basis for answering T or F, or he may be attempting to evade responding to a troubling item. Up to 50 of the 550 items can be unanswered and still not substantially lower the reliability of the MMPI[7]. The L or *Lie Score* is comprised of 15 items scattered throughout the inventory such as "I sometimes get mad," or "I have felt at times like swearing." These are items that are clear and generally socially unfavorable but which most individuals will indicate as true about themselves. Four of the 15 answered in a socially acceptable way is average for both normals and psychiatric populations. More than four lie items answered in a socially acceptable manner rather than in a realistic manner tend to reflect the test taker's motivation to place himself or herself in a more generally favorable light.

An F or *Validity Score* was derived from 65 items rarely answered by normal subjects in a deviant manner. Comprehension of the items, reading ability, apathy, or overt psychotic reactions may all contribute to an elevated F score. An elevated F score, along with elevations on the clinical scales, can be a significant finding if the examiner is attempting to assess emotional control, reality awareness, or degree of cognitive disturbance present. Changes over time on this scale are common, and previous studies have shown decreases in the elevation of F scale following therapy[8].

The K Scale is a relatively recent addition to the MMPI[9]. Its aim is to specifically assess the test-taking attitude of the subject as to suppression of or exhibition of personal defects or problems. Twenty-two items were found to be statistically significant in differentiating evasive clinical cases from more "open" individuals who would readily discuss their emotional problems.

The four validity scales, ?, L, F, and K, used individually or, more often, in relation to each other, give valuable clues as to the patient's test-taking attitudes at the time of testing. Suppose, for example, the validity scale profiles shown in Figure 4-1 were obtained on three patients.

Patient A's test-taking attitudes appear normal. Comprehension of the items (Scale F) appears adequate. Minimal overt "Fake good" efforts appear (Scale L). Moderate suppression of emotional or personality defects appear in the subject's responses (Scale K).

Patient B has evaded responding to a large number of items (Scale?). Attempts to suppress negative personality and emotional attributes appear in the patient's test responses (Scales L and K). Some elevation of F suggests the possibility of thinking and /or reasoning distortions or reading comprehension

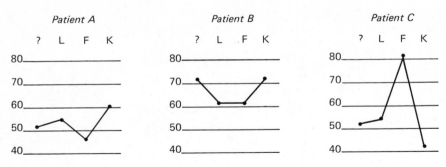

Figure 4–1.

difficulties. Later clinical scale scores may contain responses produced under conscious or unconscious efforts of patient to suppress true reactions.

Patient C has not evaded responding to the test items (?). Lowered K score suggests that little or any suppression of negative responses has occurred. The elevated F score is a source of concern. Is this elevated F score the result of poor comprehension or a reflection of the subject's tendency to "let it all hang out" (lower K, elevated F)? Patterns on later clinical scales may provide additional information, but clinical scales may be elevated due to subject's tendency to reveal greater than expected self-critical material.

The Clinical Scales. The validity scales provide some estimate of the subject's willingness to approach the task of completing the 550 items. The first three clinical scales are commonly referred to as the "Neurotic Triad" and are comprised of Scale 1 Hypochondrical, Scale 2 Depression, and Scale 3 Hysteria.

The Hypochondrisis (Hs) Scale. This scale attempts to measure abnormal concerns for bodily functions. It comprises 33 items dealing with health and physical functions. An elevated score on this scale implies overconcern, worry, and preoccupation with physical symptoms. In clinical practice, Hs elevations often accompany abnormal elevation on other clinical scales.

The Depression (D) Scale. This scale has been empirically established to measure the degree of pessimism and feelings of hopelessness. Included in this scale are items aimed at tapping the subject's preoccupation with death or suicidal thoughts. Sixty items are included on the D scale. Since feelings of depression, hopelessness, or pessimism may be a part of a neurotic or psychotic process, elevations on the D scale can also be accompanied by abnormal elevations on any of the other clinical scales.

The Hysteria (Hy) Scale. This scale was developed to differentiate those psychiatric patients suffering from conversion hysteria psychoneuroses. Sixty items are included. While many of the 60 items appear mutually contradictory, the characteristic of denial of problems, and the "smiling through clouds of gray" attitude, appear to be captured by this scale.

Configurations on the "neurotic triad" are highly significant in general medical practice. The conversion V is well known[10]. Assuming the validity scales to be within normal limits, significant elevation on Scale 1 (hypondriasis), moderate elevation on Scale 2 (depression), and abnormal elevation on Scale 3 (hysteria) have proved extremely predictive in the diagnosis and treatment of conversion hysterias showing such symptoms as low back pain without organic cause, hypertension, obesity, and vascomotor instability, as well as gastrointestinal distress. In medical practice, one often encounters patients who, no matter what is done therapeutically, continue to complain of vague sources of pain that do not respond to treatment. In such instances, MMPI findings may be extremely valuable in differential diagnosis. Depression and tension related upper G.I. tract complaints are common among elevated depression-hypochondrical patients. Ulcers are relatively rare among such males. Women with this profile exhibit a wider array of complaints, but all evidence high depression and tension. Elevated depression and hysteria individuals complain of inefficiency and inadequacy. The complaints of feeling "bottled up" and of being unable to express feelings are common. Fatigue, feelings of exhaustion without adequate organic causes, and family or marital maladjustments are also frequently observed in elevated depression-hypochondrical subjects.

The Psychopathic Deviate Scale (Pd). The 50 items included in this scale were empirically derived to measure such attitudes as disregard for social customs and mores, inability to profit from punishment, and emotional shallowness in relation to others, both in affect and in sexual relationships. Impulsiveness is also characteristically measured by the Pd scale. Elevated Pd scores suggest character deficiencies of impulse control, overindulgences in alcohol, sexual promiscuity, and problems with conformance with rules and mores in general.

The Masculinity-Feminity Scale (MF). Sixty items have been identified as significant in differentiating individuals with sexual inversions. Before labeling a subject homosexual based upon an elevated MF score, however, much additional data is necessary. In both males and females, elevated scores appear to result from high educational attainment. Clinically, elevated MF scores in normal males may indicate self-awareness, social perceptiveness, good judgment, and common sense. It would appear that the MF scale, constructed to differentiate psychiatric patients with sexual inversions, may be measuring entirely different personality characteristics in nonpsychiatric populations.

The Paranoia Scale (Pa). This scale, comprised of 40 items, attempts to measure delusions of reference and delusions of grandeur, which are included in the diagnostic concept of paranoia. Evasion, suspiciousness, and interpersonal sensitivity are areas tapped by the specific questions. Clinical practice has proven that high Pa scores in normals tend to be associated with sensitivity, worry proneness, sentimentality, peacefulness, and "softheartedness."

The Psychasthenia Scale (Pt). This scale was derived to differentiate obsessive-compulsive psychoneurotic patterns, including abnormal fears, difficulties in concentration, guilt feelings, and vacillation in decisionmaking. Forty-eight questions comprise the Pt Scale.

The Schizophrenic Scale (Sc). Seventy-five items were found to differentiate patients suffering from some form of schizophrenia from other psychiatric groups and from normals. Items dwell on social alienation, peculiarities of taste, feelings of persecution, poor family relationships, and shallowness of affect. With nonpsychiatric subjects, elevated Sc subjects are seen as prone to worry, self-dissatisfied, self-conscious, and immature.

The Manic Scale (Ma). Twenty-eight items successfully differentiate hypomanic psychiatric patients. Overactivity, emotional excitement, and flight of ideas are areas examined by the questions on the Ma scale. High Ma normal subjects are described as sociable, enthusiastic, prone to high ingestion of alcohol, and having a high energy and activity level.

The Social Interversion Scale (Si). This final clinical scale aims at differentiating social introversion, the inability to function in social settings, self-depreciatory attitudes, sensitivities, and worries concerning the subject's inability to interact with others. In normal subjects, elevated Si scores are associated with modesty, shyness, sensitivity, and lack of striving for social contacts.

Summary

A brief description of each of the MMPI's scales has been provided as originally conceived by the authors in 1940. Since its inception, applications of the MMPI in clinical settings have advanced beyond the efforts to classify individuals into one or more of the ten clinical categories. From the brief descriptions provided, the reader can seek how abnormal elevations on the psychopathic deviate scale and the manic scale would be a most common profile in delinquency, alchoholism, and other antisocial behaviors. Psychoneuroses will likely show abnormal elevations on hypochondriasis, depression, hysteria, and psychasthenia scales separately, but more often in combinations with each other. The analysis of the total profile of the MMPI's 14 scales and the interactions of combinations of scales is the task of a skilled psychologist. As more psychologists and physicians work together in rendering general medical care, the possibilities are enormous for further research into the personality/behavioral aspects of certain specific diseases; the personality/behavioral changes as a result of debilitating disease or injury; and the reduction of anxiety and tension with varying therapeutic procedures.

References

1. See Hathaway, Starke R., and McKinley, J. Charnley. A Multiphasic Personality Schedule: I. Construction of the Schedule. *Journal of Personality* 10 (1940):249–54; Hathaway, Starke R., and McKinley, J. Charnley. III. The Measurement of Symptomatic Depression. *Journal of Personality* 14(1942): 73–84; Hathaway, Starke R., and McKinley, J. Charnley. *The Minnesota Multiphasic Personality Inventory Manual, Revised*. New York: The Psychological Corporation, 1951.

2. Pearson, John S., and Swensen, Wendell M. *A User's Guide to the Mayo Clinic Automated MMPI Program*. New York: The Psychological Corporation, 1967.

3. Kamman, G.R., and Kram, C. Value of Psychometric Examinations In Medical Diagnosis and Treatment. *Journal of The American Medical Association* 158(1955):555–60.

4. Woodworth, R.S., and House, S.D. *Woodworth-House Mental Hygiene Inventory*. Chicago: C.H. Stoelting Co., 1928.

5. Bell, Hugh M. *The Adjustment Inventory*. Stanford, Calif.: Stanford University Press, 1934.

6. Bernreuter, R.G. *Personality Inventory*. Stanford, Calif.: Stanford University Press, 1931.

7. Hathaway and McKinley, *Minnesota Multiphasic Personality Inventory Manual*.

8. Barron, F., and Leary, T.F. Changes in Psychoneurotic Patients with and without Therapy. *Journal of Consulting Psychology* 19(1955):239–45.

9. Hathaway, Starke R., and Meehl, P.E. *The K Scale for the MMPI*. New York: The Psychological Corporation, 1947.

10. Hanvik, Leo J. Some Psychological Dimensions of Low Back Pain. *Journal of Consulting Psychology* 21(1951):391–97.

5

Psychosocial Counseling/Brief Psychotherapy in General Medical Settings

During the past decade, with the pressures of cost effectiveness and the need to treat large numbers of psychiatric patients of limited financial means, many forced changes occurred in the field of psychotherapy. The community mental health movement, attempting to render services to citizens of varying social, educational, and cultural backgrounds, called attention to the highly restrictive nature of orthodox psychoanalysis. Immediately a great deal of energy was directed at developing alternative techniques, including group therapies as well as more efficient one-to-one therapeutic techniques. In the process, Franz Alexander's earlier work was rediscovered[1]. In the 1940s Alexander, an orthodox psychoanalyst trained in the Freudian tradition, began experimenting with frequency of interviews and other "traditional" techniques of psychoanalysis. Patients undergoing psychoanalysis were usually seen three to five hours per week for long periods. One underlying assumption was that in order for the patient's neurosis to be identified and ultimately "cured," a "transferrence neurosis" must be developed between patient and analyst.

In some cases, the development of a full fledged transferrence neurosis may be desirable; in others it should perhaps be avoided altogether. In some it is imperative that emotional discharge and insight take place very gradually; in others with patients whose ego strength is greater, interviews with great emotional tension may be not only harmless but highly desirable.[2]

The change in the therapist's role from a passive listener to an intervening participant with the patient was also a break from tradition, along with the manipulation of the frequency of therapeutic contacts. Even with psychiatric populations, Alexander's insights have been widely adopted and incorporated into today's psychotherapeutic practices. With general medical patients, where a problem-oriented data base on the patient has been collected, and where psychodiagnostic procedures such as the MMPI are also a part of the patient's record, the utilization of brief psychotherapeutic counseling techniques is highly appropriate.

Brief therapy is characteristically a technique which is active, focused, goal-oriented, circumscribed, warmly supportive, action-oriented, and concerned with present adaptation. Traditional therapy tends to be more passive, reflective, open-ended, and patient steered; it is oriented toward feelings, self-understanding as a prerequisite to action, and the reflections of the past in the present, with the hope that enduring behavioral modifications will emerge as a result of the prolonged exploratory collaboration of patient and therapist. In contrast, brief therapy deals with a specific problem constellation. It may aim for the resolution of a present conflict or discomfort, and its objectives indeed may be of an emergency or stopgap nature.[3]

Using such a definition and applying brief psychotherapeutic techniques to patient problems in a general medical setting calls for other specific modifications. The quest for developing insight in the patient—having the patient "understand" all the conscious and unconscious factors of his fears or concerns—must be further modified in such a setting. Through the problem-oriented work-up, particularly Step 2 (Formulation of a Problem Listing), the patient has advanced or accepted the importance of an emotional/behavioral problem to his well-being. The relationship of the emotional/behavioral problem to other problem areas may not be as well understood. Coupled with a patient-delineated emotional/behavioral problem, the MMPI results are invaluable. From the validity scales, some hypotheses can be developed prior to interviewing the patient as to his attitude toward the medical-psychological process of diagnosis—his "ego strength," his evasiveness, his efforts to place himself in a good or bad light. In most instances, MMPI results can give meaningful clues as to the nature of his personality—characteristic modes of coping with stress, impulsiveness, and ability to profit from experience. This information, available in the POMIS and MMPI *prior* to face-to-face interaction between therapist and patient, enables the therapist to judge the level of insight to be sought in brief counseling without running the risk of creating undue anxiety by probing deeply into highly charged emotional areas. Several instances of near psychotic behavior have been treated successfully, with less than five therapeutic contacts, by studiously avoiding certain areas and accentuating other areas of the patient's compensatory strengths. The rule of thumb in attempting to aid the patient in development of insight is to provide the amount necessary for the patient to better understand and cope with the particular emotional/behavioral problem for which he seeks relief. The therapist using brief therapy/counseling techniques must be content to effect immediate day-to-day results rather than concerning himself with attempting to restructure personality.

Considerable controversy exists over such a "mechanistic" concept of personality. Some personality theories hold firmly to the belief that if one symptom is treated without the uncovering and "curing" of the underlying cause, then the anxiety that caused the original symptom will merely become displaced to another symptom that might be even more detrimental to the patient. Other personality theories hold that the emotional state of an individual, like his physical well-being, follows a homeostatic pattern in which disequilibrium may be followed by efforts at adaptive equilibrium. A variety of methods are available to help the patient obtain adaptive equilibrium—insight development, catharsis, intellectualization, reassurance and support, anticipatory counseling or guidance. The adaptive equilibrium view appears to be a much more parsimonious description of the brief psychotherapeutic process in general medical settings. Confined to a brief course of treatment of less than 15 interviews, the iatrogenic problem of patient dependency upon the therapist is greatly reduced. In certain instances where the patient's history and MMPI results suggest that emotional/behavioral problems are of long standing, a mutually agreed upon number of therapeutic interviews may be scheduled. At this time progress is assessed. In clinical practice, this approach has been found to be particularly useful in attempting to deal with the obsessive-compulsive individual. With patients whose MMPI results suggest problems of impulse control and difficulty with authority, a time limiting initial agreement as to the number of contacts may also be worthwhile.

Using the patient's own statement of the emotional/behavioral problem for which aid is sought, the counselor-therapist has a tangible goal of expectation. The process of turning to another human being for help is often accompanied by feelings of helplessness, anxiety, and/or hostility. With the time restrictions of brief psychosocial counseling, the therapist must establish rapport rapidly and move into the content area of the problem. Using the MMPI results and interpreting the results to the patient in the first meeting is one technique found to be very beneficial.

Introductory Remarks to Patient

"I have your health record here and have read the list of health problems which you and Dr. S. have developed. The problem which I hope I can help you with is No. 3 which is stated as 'depression.' Would you tell me in your own words what you mean by this, the feelings, and the concerns you have?"

At this point the patient is encouraged to elaborate on the concerns, the history, the length and severity of the symptoms, and upon the problem's etiology. At an appropriate point, the therapist may interject: "You filled out the 550 item questionnaire here in the office. Perhaps you would be interested in the results and the hints that your responses suggest, particularly in line with your feelings of depression and hopelessness. Remember, we don't have any instrument that can measure you feelings as accurately as a blood test can tell you your hemoglobin count. You are the ultimate judge as to whether these results adequately describe you. If these results and my interpretations are off base, please tell me. Another thing, every individual is unique, a mixture of strengths, weaknesses, likes, dislikes. There are no 'right' or 'wrong' ways that you and I, as individuals, feel about things. So please keep this in mind.

"Your MMPI suggests that you answered the items forthrightly and did not try to paint a picture of yourself as overly adjusted or poorly adjusted. Individuals who answer these items as you have are often described by others as having symptoms associated with anxiety. Stomach distress is frequently reported, along with headaches. Women with similar responses are described by peers as being very conscientious in their work, and easily hurt by criticisms or rebuffs. With married women, many report some marital problems with their husbands. In trying to understand your problem with feelings of depression, these results give me some clue as to your personality makeup and how the particular problem, depression, relates to your normal mode of functioning. Do you feel that these observations are fairly accurate, or way off base?" At this point the patient will usually corroborate the interpretation, accentuating certain observations, downplaying others. The open and direct method of sharing with the patient the findings and hypotheses gleaned from the MMPI *in common language*, free from psychiatric and psychological jargon, has been found to be one of the most effective means of establishing early patient-therapist rapport. Thirty-eight critical items within the MMPI have been developed, bearing on some serious symptom, impulse, or experience[4]. In scoring the MMPI, deviant responses to these 38 critical items are noted and put aside for later, more intensive questioning.

After obtaining the patient's reactions to the general MMPI interpretations, the therapist has the stage structured to move on in to more sensitive areas.

"On the 550 items, there are several which I want to discuss more fully with you. You checked as 'true' the response to the statement 'I have had many strange and unusual experiences.' What was going through your mind when you checked this as 'true'?" (Other items related to sexual attitudes, fear of mental illness, etc., can be approached in the same forthright manner.)

Using the patient's responses to the MMPI, rather than "digging" into sensitive areas, appears to communicate to the patient that *his* concerns, and *his* responses are the starting point in the therapeutic process. Without such a starting point, the therapist is forced, by direct questioning and history taking, to cover a wide variety of interpersonal and attitudinal areas, often conveying to the patient that the quest for information is more important than the therapist's sensitivities to the patient. Under the press to get on with the process of helping the patient solve his immediate problem in a minimal number of interview sessions, an instrument such as the MMPI has proved invaluable.

The Phases of Psychosocial Counseling

Wolberg has broken brief psychotherapy into four stages.[5] Psychosocial counseling follows the same developmental phases.

The Supportive Phase

Stage one, the supportive phase, entails the following steps:

1. to establish as rapidly as possible a working relationship;
2. to treat the patient as a worthwhile individual no matter what his emotional state or neurotic difficulties;
3. to inspire the patient to verbalize as much as possible;
4. to avoid arguing or quarreling with the patient;
5. to communicate empathy; and
6. to convey verbally and nonverbally the confidence that the therapist can help the patient without promising a "cure."

In setting the stage for the supportive phase, the utilization of the MMPI in the manner described has proven invaluable in achieving the above six objectives.

The Apperceptive Stage

During the second stage, the therapist strives to help the individual achieve some recognition of what might be behind his particular emotional problem. Prior relationship with parents and siblings, precipitating factors, job stress, and all possible and potential factors could be incorporated into a full blown psychiatric history. Time, however, under the restrictions of brief therapy, prevents such a complete workup. Again, by utilizing the MMPI as an "ice breaker" during the supportive stage, as well as a method of helping the individual obtain some perspective as to his problem in relation to his emotional makeup, speeds this apperceptive stage, the therapist-counselor may make a judgment to not probe a potentially disruptive area of the patient's life. A 27 year old automobile salesman, who had attempted suicide at 19, received one year of inpatient psychiatric treatment following discharge from the army, and who answered "False" to the statement "My Father was a good man," is not a good candidate for aggressive questioning concerning his early childhood relationships with his father. If, in later discussion, he *voluntarily* brings up this topic, as a means of furthering his understanding of his current problem, all well and good. To use a meat ax, however, without gauging the severity and potential disruptive result of such probing behavior, is to risk not only the therapeutic outcome, but the ultimate well-being of the patient.

The Action Phase

In this stage of progress, the patient attempts to put his acquired understanding or acquired convictions into actual behavior. During this stage, even the smallest evidence of progress is labeled as success. Progressive desensitization programs, and techniques such as progressive relaxation, biofeedback, and hypnosis, have been found useful in aiding the patient to move into the action stage. The adage "Nothing succeeds like success," is crucial at this stage. The support and reinforcement of the therapist as well as of members of his family may require the therapist's interaction with others on behalf of the patient.

The Integrative Stage

The last stage is when the patient, over long periods of time, integrates his newer modes of behavior into his every day behavior. The brief therapist–psychosocial counselor usually does not have the privilege of observing this firsthand, and must usually develop some form of followup to finally observe the patient's progress into this fourth and final stage. In a general medical setting, the psychotherapist-counselor may ask the physician, in subsequent medical contacts, to assess the patient's progress and subsequent behavior. When the patient is terminated from brief counseling, three-month and six-month follow-up visits are ideal. In some instances, notes to the physician may be included in the problem notes, such as: "Ask the patient about success in school"; or "Is the patient still on speaking terms with mother-in-law?" Certain critical behaviors can indicate to the psychotherapist-counselor how well the patient continues to function.

Summary

This chapter has attempted to convey the style and techniques of setting the stage for rendering brief psychotherapy/psychosocial counseling in a general medical setting. The author, having worked in outpatient psychiatric clinics, inpatient psychiatric settings, and as a consultant to comprehensive community mental health centers, is convinced that counseling, provided as a natural adjunct of general medical care, is the method of choice. Stigma problems that the patient may suffer from being referred to a mental health provider are greatly reduced. Combining the complete medical and psychological records of the patient proves invaluable to both the physician and the psychotherapist-counselor. Perhaps most importantly, by the physician and psychologist working together in continuous contact around the patient's problems, an ongoing interchange can occur that reduces the dichotomy between soma and psyche, which cannot occur in exclusively mental health or medical settings. In the case material contained in later chapters, the interchange and interaction of the physician and psychologist around the patient's problems is amply demonstrated.

Throughout this book, the terms "brief psychotherapy" and "brief counseling" are used interchangeably. When one examines the definitions that attempt to differentiate psychotherapy versus counseling, one of the key points of demarcation lies in the type of patient receiving services. Psychotherapy is generally applied to services rendered to individuals with a diagnosed psychological or psychiatric condition. Counseling, on the other hand, generally conveys the process of providing services to nonpsychiatric populations in an effort to solve more "normal" problems—i.e., educational counseling and marriage counseling.

With general medical patients seeking primary health care, both psychiatric/psychological and "normal" adjustment problems are encountered, as the case histories in the chapters to follow demonstrate. To convey both psychotherapeutic and counseling activities, which are dictated by the needs of general medical patients, the term "psychosocial counseling" appears more descriptive, hence the title of this book—*Psychosocial Counseling in General Medical Practice*.

References

1. Alexander, Franz, and French, Thomas M. *Psychoanalytic Therapy*. New York: Ronald Press Company, 1946, 1974 p. 46. © 1946, 1974 The Ronald Press Company, New York. Reprinted by permission.

2. Ibid.

3. Barton, Harvey H. *Brief Therapies*. New York: Behavioral Publications, 1971, pp. 8–9. Reprinted by permission.

4. Hellman, L.I. Appendix G. Critical Items. In Dahlstrom, W. Grant, and Welsh, George S. *An MMPI Handbook*. Minneapolis, Minn.: University of Minnesota Press, 1960, pp. 434–35.

5. Wolberg, Lewis. Methodology in Short-Term Therapy. *American Journal of Psychiatry* 122(1961):135–40.

6

"Style of Life" Counseling/
Psychotherapy

In the course of relating to a patient seeking relief from a specific complaint, conducting the necessary physical and laboratory workup and interacting with the patient in redefining health problem areas, the physician's role as a teacher-educator is perhaps more important than as a dispenser of medical cures. In Chapter 3 reference has been made to the changing patterns in health problems and in the rendering of health care. In the early 1900s the major diseases were for the most part singularly caused. Today, seeking "the single cause" for metabolic disorders such as diabetes mellitus, or for the pathology of arteriosclerosis, cancer, schizophrenia and many types of arthritis, is to utilize a simplistic approach that does not conform to current research findings.

Diseases of the circulatory system, the chief cause of death in the United States today, provides the major example. Table 6-1 shows the percent of all deaths from coronary heart disease in 1967.

The cardiovascular diseases, including all forms, are responsible for more than one-third of all deaths among persons under 65 years of age. What is known concerning the preventive aspects of coronary heart disease? A variety of "risk factors" have been identified. Serum lipids and diet, including elevated serum triglycerides, cholesterol, and saturated fats, have been isolated as having a positive statistical relationship with occurrence of heart disease.[1] Overweight and obesity are known to be frequently associated with certain coronary heart diseases.[2] Hypertension, in epidemologic studies, is a known correlate of many coronary conditions. A significant relationship between cigarette smoking and increased risk of developing coronary artery disease has been demonstrated. Diabetes mellitis and impaired glucose tolerance have been shown to be statistically related to arteriosclerotic disease.[3] Sedentary living, psychological stresses, and genetic constitutional factors have also been observed as correlates to coronary disease.

If one approaches coronary disease in the tradition of the 1900s, which of these potential causes will we try to eradicate? Which is *the* cause? Which one of this array of potential causal factors will we focus upon and attempt to educate our patients to avoid? Approaching the prevention of coronary disease as a

Table 6–1
Percent of All Deaths for Coronary Heart Disease by Age, Sex, and Color: United States, 1967

Color and sex	Age groups							
	Under 25	25–34	35–44	45–54	55–64	65–74	75–84	85 and over
White male	0.28	5.28	26.48	39.41	42.24	42.35	41.84	42.21
White female	0.23	3.03	8.01	15.27	26.64	37.19	41.01	42.06
Nonwhite male	0.37	4.99	13.78	21.38	27.22	29.49	32.35	34.28
Nonwhite female	0.33	5.36	10.18	17.31	24.01	29.39	32.77	35.61
All	0.29	4.70	17.85	28.98	35.49	39.09	40.85	41.72

Source: From Sartwell, Maxcy-Rosneau Preventive Medicine and Public Health, 10th edition, 1973, p. 462. Courtesy of Appleton-Century-Crofts, Publishing Division of Prentice-Hall, Inc.

complex multiplicity-caused illness complicates the preventive efforts of the physician in attempting to educate or reeducate his patient.

In order to do an adequate job in educating his patient, the physician must keep abreast of current research efforts. Clinically, based upon his intimate knowledge of the patient as a person, as a biological entity, and as a social and psychological personality, the physician must translate these current scientific findings and hypotheses into meaning for the patient. This process of introducing to the patient current causal theories of disease and relating these causal factors both intellectually and emotionally to the meaningful life areas of the patient, is a most difficult undertaking. The process is, however, "primary prevention."

The face-to-face interaction in which the goal is primary prevention has been labeled "style of life" counseling/psychotherapy, for want of a better term. When psychological characterisitics of the patient are included in the total diagnostic physical workup, rather than complicating the process of education-reeducation, the process is actually made easier. The process of obtaining some indication of the patient's temperament, his concerns and over-concerns, along with a suggestion as to how he characteristically reacts to stress, addressed in Chapter 4, provides guidelines as to techniques, approaches, and the level of importance the counselor will attach to the changes needed in the lifestyle of the patient. Even with the added insights provided by psychodiagnostic techniques, the ultimate outcome depends upon the acceptance and behavioral changes *within* the patient and cannot be completely predicted. On occasion, when educational-reeducational efforts are attempted, the patient may evidence immediate hostility and resentment toward the physician or psychologist. Remarks such as "You sound like my wife, who has been nagging me for years to cut down on my smoking!" or "I didn't ask you to do a reconstruction job on me, merely treat this pain!" indicate that the patient's receptivity to suggestions of a primary preventive nature has not developed sufficiently for the counselor-therapist to make headway. This is a risk that is constantly present, yet, for the patient to be a full partner in his health care, he must begin to accept such suggestions as the best clinical judgments for his future well-being.

A common phenomenon that occurs when the physician attempts primary prevention with a seemingly reluctant patient is the delayed response. After apparently rejecting efforts at primary prevention, where certain modifications of the patient's lifestyle have been suggested to reduce chances of a health problem occurrence in the future, the patient may grow to accept such suggestions. The time interval may be weeks, months, years, or perhaps never. Such is the calculated risk that the primary physician must accept if the patient is to be perceived as a full partner in his own health care and if the health provider sees his role not only as an ameliorator of immediate health problems but as a provider of counsel to prevent recurrence or to avoid future problems. The case examples provided demonstrate successes, failures, and instances in which the outcome is still unknown.

The Case of James

James is a 34-year-old full-time insurance salesman for a midwestern multiline insurance company. Over 2,400 agents are employed and many administrative opportunities exist, for which the patient is studying to advance within the company's structure. James is married and there are three children, ages nine, eight, and six. His hobbies include scuba diving, and all forms of outdoor sports. There is no family history of rheumatic fever or cardiovascular disease, but there is a diabetic tendency in the maternal lineage. His reason for seeking out-patient treatment is a "feeling of tiredness" for the past several months. Prior medical contacts are recorded for hernia repair, vasectomy, and for a giant cell tumor removal on his big toe.

Physical and Laboratory Workup

Physical examination revealed a Caucasian male, five feet, seven inches tall, weighing 197 pounds, approximately 20 percent overweight; blood pressure was recorded at 134/98, urine analysis and blood chemistry studies reveal abnormally high glucose readings. For over 15 years the patient has smoked two packs of cigarettes per day. During the past year the patient has suffered puffy ankles. He has limited exercise except on occasional weekends when he enjoys his hobby, scuba diving. He works under considerable pressure, drinks more than five cups of coffee per day and enjoys at least two cocktails per day in the course of his work and social activities.

Because of frequent 10- to 14-hour workdays during the past several years, he and his wife have "grown apart." In the view of the patient, his wife is more "home and children" oriented, while he is trying to get ahead financially.

Since his discharge from the army ten years ago, the patient has noticed hearing difficulties and had been told, while in the army, that some nerve damage was present that might cause hearing problems in later life.

Medical Problem Profile

In interpreting these findings to the patient, the following problems were jointly rank ordered:

1. history of diabetes and borderline diabetic condition, likely one source of "feeling of tiredness";
2. hearing deficit;
3. excessive smoking—probably also contributing to precipitating reason for seeking medical help;

4. marital difficulties—growing differences between patient and wife and less mutual enjoyment.

Personality Profile

On the MMPI, the profile given in Figure 6-1 was obtained.

MMPI results suggest an individual who has tendencies to overreact, difficulties with impulse control, and perhaps exhibits excessives in drinking, merrymaking, and, in general, "acting-out" behavior. In dealings with others, one might expect the patient to be a lively conversationalist, fluent, lacking in self-consciousness, and typifying the successful salesman. In answering specific items, the patient indicates that his sex life is unsatisfactory, that he is concerned about sex matters and has used alcohol excessively. Statistically, individuals with similar MMPI profiles complain frequently of tension and fatigue but experience hypomanic periods. Poor family adjustment and problems associated with sexual adjustment are frequent complaints.

Discussion

The MMPI results, integrated with James' medical findings, suggest that his style of life is probably the key to ameliorating present complaints and to heading off future difficulties. With his personality makeup, merely suggesting dietary restrictions, giving up smoking, or curtailing his work habits would have little, if any, impact. As a calculated risk, the physician and psychologist decided that the psychologist should attempt counseling with James in an effort to enlist his understanding and commitment. As a result, a "one shot" consultation was scheduled. James' medical findings were reiterated, plus the MMPI results, as described in Chapter 4. In the course of interpreting the personality facets, both the positive and negative aspects of his MMPI findings were included. After an initial reaction of guardedness, James stated that the problem with his wife was much more severe than initially revealed. His wife is presently seeking marital counseling and is contemplating the future with or without James.

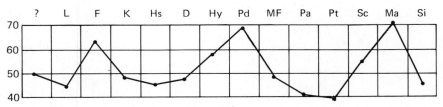

Figure 6-1.

Despite direct urgings by his wife, James has avoided accepting that marital counseling might help, and has begun work longer hours, have more social drinks, let his eyes wander to sexually attractive coworkers, and in general, has avoided the immediate marital problem by throwing himself more into his job and into training courses aimed at advancing him within his insurance organization.

The interrelationship between his borderline diabetic condition, his symptoms of tiredness, and his overindulgences in smoking, alcohol, and work habits, as well as his home tensions, were interpreted to him. As to the solutions of these multiple problems, the psychologist freely admitted that he did not know where to start in rectifying the situation. Yet, out of concern for James as a patient, and out of a desire to provide him with the most complete understanding of his present and future health needs, it was felt that these matters should be discussed with him. At the conclusion of the hour interview, James was asked to mull these things over and decide what he wanted to do. No further appointments were made, but James was encouraged to contact the office if he felt any desire to discuss these problems further.

Six months after this "one shot" effort, James has not returned for discussions about these specific problems. On one occasion, he sought medical help because of eye inflammation that appeared to be the result of eye strain. During his contact, upon leaving the consultation room, he said to the physician, "Tell Dr. H. that I am going to the marriage counselor, not that it's going to do any good!" Blood pressure was 134/86 and weight was recorded as 191 pounds.

At his writing, the effort to enlist James' cooperation in his health problems is still a moot question. Whether such primary preventive efforts will produce results may never be completely answered. In any event, the effort has not interfered with his returning to the office for routine medical care. In the words of Hippocrates, he might not have been helped but he has not apparently been hurt by these efforts. Statistically, with James' high profile on many of the risk factors currently held to be related to coronary disease, unless changes do occur in his lifestyle, the probabilities are high that he will be one of the victims of coronary disease before he reaches age 65.

The Case of Gene

This 44-year-old rancher was referred to the physician from a medical colleague in a small rural community. He is married to an elementary school teacher and there are four children, ages seven to 20. Gene has been active in civic and community activities up until the past year. No known family history of rheumatic fever or cardiovascular disease. His mother and grandfather died young of unknown causes; the grandfather developed blindness before his death.

Gene sought treatment because of kidney stones and suspected diabetes.

Three months prior to referral, he had undergone a vasectomy recommended by his family physician at home. He reports that he healed poorly and suffered progressive feelings of nervousness. Two weeks prior to referral, he passed a kidney stone with considerable pain. Patient was admitted to the general hospital and disgnostic tests were begun.

Physical and Laboratory Findings

Physically, Gene is a well-developed, slightly overweight 44-year-old white male who appears somewhat ruddy and balding. He appears in good general health. His blood pressure is 134/80. His chest, heart, and lungs are all normal. Blood studies reveal normal count and urine reveals no evidence of sugar or albumen. Repeated glucose tolerance tests and insulin levels suggest delayed release of insulin, strongly supporting the diagnosis of early diabetes mellitis. As to his emotional feelings of tension and anxiety, a neurologic examination revealed no abnormalities and the neurologist concluded that Gene appeared to be suffering anxiety attacks that may or may not be triggered by variations in his blood sugar.

Medical Problem Profile

After obtaining all consultant reports, laboratory findings, X-ray, etc., the following list of health problems was developed between Gene and his attending physician.

1. Diabetes mellitis: probably accounting for lack of healing, tiredness, and a portion of his nervousness.
2. Kidney stones: G.I. series revealed no other stones of any magnitude, but periodic X-rays will be scheduled.
3. Nervousness: feelings of tension and anxiety, while related to problems 1 and 2 above, probably are a separate problem and should be treated as such.
4. Periodic attacks of Gout.
5. Minor rectal bleeding.

Personality Profile

The MMPI results obtained from Gene while in the hospital are given in Figure 6-2. Males showing similar MMPI configurations often demonstrate somatic overconcerns with little demonstrable physical pathology. In the face of stress, they will often use physical difficulties to solve emotional problems. The con-

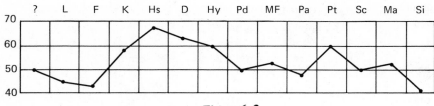

Figure 6–2.

clusion drawn from Gene's MMPI was that he is an essentially normal individual; however, he has some psychoneurotic tendencies centering around overconcern with somatic functioning, probably of long standing. Responses to individual items suggest fears of losing his mind, along with chronic anxiety.

Discussion

Whether the causes or the result of diabetes mellitis, Gene's emotional state had to be considered in his overall treatment. In interviewing Gene in the hospital, he stated that he had never experienced anything like this before. He attributes the start of his difficulty to the vasectomy performed five months ago. In discussing this, he reports he had this done at the urging of his physician to prevent further pregnancies by his wife. He admits to having been quite frightened about the prospect of a vasectomy, but after reading a pamphlet that told of a vasectomy as "a minor operation with no after pain and complete recovery in two or three days," he finally consented to the operation. Five days after the operation, he and his wife vacationed at Las Vegas and he returned home "feeling like the Devil." When asked what this meant, he finally related that he was depressed, agitated, and fearful that his "manhood" had been interfered with. At the time of passing the kidney stone, the precipitating reason for referral, Gene admitted that in spite of the pain, he was greatly relieved because he now had a physical reason to explain his "feeling like the Devil." Gene's preoccupation with his health problems had totally interfered with his role in his home community as county commissioner.

Gene related how his mother and a favorite uncle had died slow and painful deaths in his early youth. He admits to a deep-rooted fear of being physically incapacitated and says this fear has been plaguing him for several months. The MMPI results were interpreted to him and the interpretation given that these physical and emotional reactions, all occurring in close succession to each other, could account for his "feeling like the Devil." Encouragement and reassurance were given, particularly stressing the point that none of the physical difficulties would be incapacitating or interfere with his style of life. Gene returned home and, in subsequent contacts, reports that tinges of apprehension and anxiety still occur occasionally, but such episodes are of short duration and do not interfere with his enjoyment or work obligations. Back home in his rural community, he continues to extol the fine medical care he received and has been the source of many referrals of friends and relatives.

The Case of Cora

Cora is a 44-year-old matron, the mother of three children, ranging in age from 15 to 20. The older son is in college. The second child, a daughter, is a senior in high school. Cora's husband is 54, is employed by a large corporation, and is currently unhappy with his work. He is thinking of an early retirement. Cora's social activities have centered around a few close friends. There is no family history of cardiovascular disease or diabetes. The patient had previously required low back surgery five years ago. Four years ago a total hysterectomy was performed as a result of endometriosis. Cora's reason for seeking medical care was the occurrence, some two weeks ago, of a small hemorrhoid. Cora states that she has suffered from a spastic colon for the past several years.

Physical and Laboratory Findings

Physical examination revealed blood pressure of 120/80, weight 124 pounds, height five feet, four inches. Mobility is impaired as a result of back surgery, patient can bend within 12 inches of the floor. A left thrombosed hemorrhoid is present. Sigmoidoscopy was performed, with negative findings. Blood studies were normal, including estrogen level.

Medical Problem Profile

Together with Cora, the following problems were identified and rank ordered in priority.

1. Minor hemmorrhoids probably will respond to external treatment; no surgery required at this time.
2. "Spastic colon," which appears to be related to periodic stress.
3. Loss of confidence and accompanying feelings of depression.
4. Secondary arthritis in spine with seasonal pain.

Personality Profile

Cora's MMPI profile is shown in Figure 6-3.
   Shy, self-distrusting, suffering from social alienation are descriptions of women showing profiles similar to Cora's. Depression, particularly the "smiling"

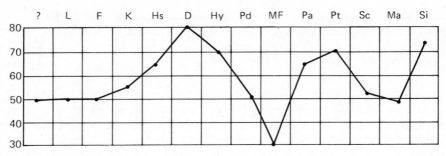

Figure 6–3.

variety, might be suspected and may have existed for a number of years. Under stress, in addition to feelings of self-depreciation, the patient will likely "somatize" her anxieties.

Discussion

Combining the findings of Cora's medical and psychological assessment, it was felt that Cora might be helped if she could be encouraged to break out of her social isolating shell. A conference with the psychologist was scheduled.

The MMPI results were interpreted to Cora, who substantiated that her social shyness had been a source of pain since her childhood. During her early married years, she wrapped herself up in the care and upbringing of her children. When her oldest child left home to attend college, she began to anticipate and worry about how life would be when ultimately all her children were gone from home. Her spastic colon attacks have been more frequent and severe since the oldest son left home to attend college. Her interests and hobbies have always been centered around the home (baking bread, sewing, knitting, etc.) and in her present state of depression give her no pleasure. Cora has never been able to communicate her emotional feelings to her husband for fear he would not understand. When asked what she would like to do, even in her wildest daydreams, she told of having taken typing in high school and wondered if she could ever bring her skills up to a level where she could be employed part-time. Her next door neighbor had been encouraging her to attend a church-sponsored self-betterment course, which Cora wanted to attend, but felt afraid because she did not know the people.

A discussion then took place about a woman's changing role, particularly when her children reach maturity. Cora was asked if her anticipation of loneliness after the children leave was not one of her major concerns. She readily agreed, but voiced fear that she did not have the ability or strength to change. The one-hour session ended with the therapist encouraging Cora to set as a goal for herself attending the church self-betterment course during the coming week. An appointment was made for Cora to return to the therapist to discuss her experiences in three weeks.

Cora returned and actually glowed with the enjoyment and encouragement she had received from the church group, which had scheduled weekly meetings. In the self-betterment course, cybernetics was strongly extolled. Cora had become deeply involved in the readings and brought along a paper that she had prepared for class presentation. One quotation: "One point I will remember daily is my disturbed feelings—anger, fear, anxiety, insecurity—are caused by my own response, not by external things. So often before I believed differently, that my disturbed feelings were the other person's fault but now this is not so; it is my own response which determines the outcome of my feelings." Cora was complimented on the content as well as the neatness of the typing. She reported that she is going to take a typing refresher course at the local high school two evenings per week. Encouragement and praise were given Cora and an appointment made to see her in a month.

In subsequent monthly contacts, Cora reported that she completed her typing course and has obtained a part-time job. Her outlook, and her physical and emotional health, have changed drastically. Her style of life, previously centered in her home around her children and their needs, has been altered and expanded. Cora and her husband have a better relationship, and the void created by children growing up and leaving seems to have been partially filled.

Summary

Style of life counseling is the health provider's attempt to apply theories of causality to the future well-being of one patient. Changes in behavior, in habits of long duration, and in emotional and psychological adjustments are often involved. As such, immediate results are not often evident, but may be delayed over months and years. Instances do occur, however, that suggest that, depending upon the patient's readiness to accept alterations of behavior at that time, significant changes in patient behavior can occur. In any event, if the process of offering style of life counseling to a patient conveys the health practitioner's concern for the future health and well-being of the patient, then the patient likely will harbor no ill will or resentment toward the doctor. After all, responsibility for style of life changes rests squarely with the patient, but on occasion the patient does not want to hear or accept this. In such instances, such preventive efforts are stored away in the hope that an opportune time will arrive in the future.

References

1. Lilienfeld, Abraham M. Diseases of the Circulatory System. In *Maxcy-Rosneau Preventive Medicine and Public Health,* 10th edition, Philip E. Sartwell, ed. New York: Appleton-Century-Crofts, 1973, pp. 461–76.

2. Report of Intersociety Commission for Heart Disease Resources. Primary Prevention of the Arteriosclerotic Diseases. *Circulation* 42(1970):53.

3. Epstein, F.H. Hyperglycemia: A Risk Factor in Coronary Heart Disease. *Circulation* 36(1967):609.

7

Depression and Grief in General
Medical Practice

Depression, as a primary health problem or as a secondary reaction to almost any medical and/or psychiatric problem, is one of the most common problems in any health setting. Cross has tabulated the most commonly seen acute and long term problems observed in a general medical practice in a small town during a six-month period.[1] Table 7-1 contains his findings of the number of patients exhibiting these problems.

The high incidence of emotional/behavioral diagnoses in general practice, and particularly of depression, can be clearly seen from these diagnoses.

Depression has been described in terms of its paradoxes. There is a wide gap between the depressed person's image of self and objective facts. A successful business man becomes fearful that he will not provide for his family, a beautiful woman feels that she is ugly, an acclaimed scholar feels he is stupid. Patients holding to such self-debasing ideas are not easily swayed by evidence or logical reasoning to the contrary. Depression, described as melancholia over 2,000 years ago by the Greeks, continues to be a puzzling clinical syndrome as well as presenting major unresolved issues regarding its nature, classification, and etiology. Beyond such clinical concerns, there are everyday concerns of feelings of depression, sense of failure, and "blue" periods which universally occur in normal individuals. When does a "blue period" become severe enough to warrant the diagnosis of depression? Is depression a type of reaction to real or anticipated stress or is it a distinct disease entity? Is depression biologically caused or psychosocially caused? What about grief reactions, the result of the death of a spouse; is this a normal depressive reaction to a sense of loss, or is it qualitatively different from the clinical syndrome called depression? These and many other questions concerning this mood disorder remain unanswered. According to Kline, depression is recognized as a contributing factor to more human suffering than any other single disease or condition affecting mankind.[2]

Subjectively, the writer has found that the concept of "elasticity" helps in making judgments as to severity, normal versus abnormal, and illness versus normal mood swing that the clinician is often forced to make. Accepting the fact that extraneous circumstances occur that can create loneliness, self-despair, self-debasement, and self-blame, the critical element in this process is the

49

Table 7–1

Frequency of Encounters by Diagnosis, January–June 1971

1. Depression	307
2. Conversion reaction	306
3. Obesity	261
4. Bronchitis, acute	247
5. Anxiety	232
6. Hearing loss, u, c.	200
7. HCVD	191
8. Diabetes mellitis	182
9. Upper respiratory infections	170
10. Otitis media	168
11. Pharynigitis, nonstrep	143
12. Strep pharynigitis	139
13. Minor trauma	131
14. Abdominal pain, u, c.	126
15. Bronchopneumonia	113
16. L-S Back pain, U, c.	110
17. Situational reaction (adult)	110
18. Hemorrhoids	109
19. Respiratory flu	103
20. ASHD	98

Source: Harold D. Cross, *The Problem-Oriented System in Private Practice in a Small Town.*
In *Applying The Problem-Oriented System.* Edited by H. Kenneth Walker and J. Willishurst.
Baltimore: Williams and Wilkins, 1973, pg.-159. Reprinted by permission.

disequilibrium-equilibrium balance which, over time, the individual strives to recover. In a short book called *Good Grief*, the developmental stages of normal
grief reaction are described in detail.[3] After stages of shock, disbelief, self-
pity, and anger, a reintegration or equilibrium is finally achieved in which the
sufferer concludes that life must go on. This ability to reintegrate, to obtain
some semblance of homeostasis, to "pick up the pieces" from the past and to
look more to the present and the future, represents a sort of resilience, "an elasticity," bending with current trials and tribulations, but ultimately returning
to a tolerable mode of existence. Using such a concept of "elasticity" helps the
practitioner in his judgments as to the normalcy-abnormalcy decision that must
be made if a treatment plan is to be formulated to help the patient. Current
societal practices surrounding death appear to be calculated to reduce the ultimate realization that a person has actually died. The presence of a nurse at the
funeral home, the reference to the deceased as "sleeping," as "passed away," the
avoidance of the word "death," all tend to prolong and delay the ultimate
realization that the person is no longer present and living in a physical sense.
Consequently, the griever does not have an immediate opportunity to accept his
ultimate and final loss and to work out his normal grief reaction. In many
"depressions" encountered among general medical patients, the feelings of loss
and of self-blame associated with the death of a loved one in the past, *which
have never been "worked through",* are often the source of immediate depression.

Accepting the judgmental factors that must be made around the label of depression and further accepting the pervasive nature of negative mood swings in most human beings, the following definition is offered. Depression is defined pragmatically in terms of the following characteristics:

1. a prolonged change or alteration from the typical or usual outlook on life, with emphasis on sadness, loneliness, apathy;
2. a negative self-concept, including self-blame and self-chastisement, which does not conform to objective realities;
3. regressive and self-punitive wishes, including the desire to escape, hide, or die;
4. vegetative changes, insomnia, loss of libido, weight loss;
5. changes in activity level, including psychomotor retardation or agitation.[4]

In studying the content of complaints by individuals suffering from clinically diagnosed depressive states, Cassidy, Flanagan, and Spellman found that complaints fall in six categories:[5]

1. Psychological (58 percent): "depressed," "nothing to look forward to," "no interest," "deeply discouraged," "can't remember things," "all mixed up," "very unhappy," etc.
2. Localized medical complaints (18 percent): "head hurts," "pressure in chest," "urinating frequently," "upset stomach," etc.
3. Generalized medical complaints (11 percent): "tired," "exhausted," "feel all in," "can't do work because of lack of strength," "trembling," etc.
4. Medical and psychological (2 percent): "get scared to death and can't breathe," "have no power, arms feel weak," "I can't work," etc.
5. Medical, general and local (2 percent).
6. No complaints (9 percent).

Listening to the patient's own semantic description of his physical, emotional, and intellectual capabilities reveals the clues from which one gauges the presence or absence of depressive feeling tones, as well as an estimate as to the depth, severity, and length of such an emotional state. A depression can be the first sign of an impending psychotic reaction. A depression can denote the slippage of neurotic control patterns or may appear as a stage in a normal reaction to grief. In many ways, depression is analogous to an elevated temperature— it signifies that something is wrong. To therefore respond to the depression alone, without making an effort to determine if such a depression is primary or secondary, is to miss many of the nuances of what a depression on the part of the patient is actually communicating.

In the chapter dealing with the MMPI (Chapter 4), the D or depression scale was described as a most sensitive instrument in detecting depressive feelings of the patient at the time of testing. By the configuration of D in relation to the other nine clinical scales, inferences can be drawn as to whether the depressive aspects of a patient's discomfort are the primary source of his discomfort or suggest deeper personality problems. In studies comparing the patient's progress and improvement in overcoming a depressive state, the MMPI, with repeated administration, has been found to be one of the best existing instruments for tracking the progress of the patient's depressive state. The case records selected for inclusion in this chapter illustrate examples of depression as a primary causal factor in general medical practice. In following chapters on neurotic and psychotic reactions, in almost every clinical instance depression is an accompanying symptom.

The Case of Diane

This 36-year-old housewife and mother was born in Kansas, where she attended the state university and obtained an elementary teacher's certificate. She taught school for eight years, then met and married a physician, who had been married previously. Two children, ages seven and nine, resulted from this union. There is a family history of breast cancer in the maternal grandmother, but no known history of rheumatic fever or diabetes. The reason for contact was to obtain a complete physical. Since she had never had a problem-oriented workup, this was undertaken.

Physical and Laboratory Findings

The patient is a petite five foot, two inch, Caucasian weighing 105 pounds. Blood pressure was 110/70. Blood studies revealed a borderline white blood count. Endocrine levels were in the normal range. A glucose tolerance series revealed no suggestions of abnormal functioning. Physical examination revealed vaginitis which appeared to be confined to left labia minora with some cervix involvement.

Medical Problem Profile

In collaboration with Diane, a listing of present and anticipated health problems was developed and rank ordered, according to the concerns of the patient.

1. Social dissociation: Separation from husband has occurred during past month. Husband moved out of house, leaving patient with responsibilities for children, bills, and household upkeep.
2. Nervous G.I. tract: While not active at this time, patient has a tendency toward "upset stomach" following prolonged periods of stress.

3. Kidney stones: Not a problem at this time, but patient had previously been told that stones existed and might some day cause trouble (upper G.I. study underway).
4. Recurrent vaginitis: Appears to be Herpes Type II. Previously has responded to Mycostatin and Vanobid and silver nitrate.
5. Periodic attacks of rheumatism/bursitis: No problems at present but should be kept in mind.
6. Family history of breast cancer (Annual mammography routine being established).

Personality Profile

On the MMPI, the profile shown in Figure 7-1 was obtained.

The results suggest that Diane attempted to answer the questions honestly. There is a suggestion that at the time of taking the MMPI, Diane's defenses are at a minimum and she feels relatively defenseless. Two peaks occur, on depression and social introversion. The elevation on social introversion suggests a modest, shy, self-effacing individual who might be described by close acquaintances as kind, affectionate, soft-hearted, and sentimental. This is not the response of an individual who strives for social contacts. The "style of life" suggested by the elevated social introversion scale has probably been a characteristic of Diane since maturity.

Superimposed upon the "style of life" there appears to be depression. While within the normal limits, medical patients with elevated D scores complain of depression with some physical symptomology. Responses to critical items suggest problems in attitudes toward sex and feelings of tension and anxiety most of the time.

Discussion

Combining the medical and physiological material, it would appear that Diane's problem list has several elements suggesting emotional reactions to stress. Her

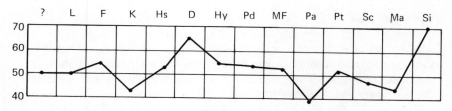

Figure 7-1.

"nervous stomach," and perhaps the recurrent vaginitis, could be indirectly associated with her marital difficulty. It was felt that with her present state of relative defenselessness, and her previous difficulty in establishing a workable doctor-patient relationship, she should be seen periodically, and help was offered for problem 1.

An appointment was scheduled and her MMPI results interpreted. Her shyness has always been a problem, combined with fear of what others might think of her. One month after her husband's departure she continues to "put up the front" that he is home and things are normal. In order to do this, she avoids church, or any contacts with neighbors or friends. This withdrawal solution to her problems would be expected from her elevated social introversion score; however, it was interpreted to Diane that this approach would not solve the problem currently facing her. She was encouraged to seek legal advice and urged to keep in touch with both the physician and psychologist. One week later she called the psychologist to say that in mulling over the problem, she had decided to tell her parents of her marital difficulties, and to go and visit them for several weeks. Since school was not in session, a prolonged visit would not disrupt the children's schedule.

Upon her return a month later, she was much more relaxed. She could now express hostility toward her husband and was actively participating with her lawyer to obtain an adequate and equitable settlement. She stated that she knew it was not good for her to withdraw socially and emotionally, for it caused her to live through her children and to satisfy her needs vicariously. She had inquired about reinstatement of her teaching certificate and is planning to take required refresher courses.

Over the past two years Diane has continued to maintain contact. Her husband has elected to seek psychiatric counseling and is attempting a reconciliation. Diane continues to force herself to participate in activities outside the home and has adopted a philosophical attitude toward her marriage. In the future, she will continue to contact her physician and psychologist when she needs support or when she needs help in coping with decisions that must be made. Her husband has indicated some surprise in Diane's new lifestyle. She no longer retreats when she becomes hurt in her interactions with him.

The Case of Julius

This 70-year-old ex-mechanic and ex-rancher retired from full-time work five years ago, but continued to work part-time until six months ago. He has been married for 30 years to a 59-year-old woman with two children by a previous marriage. There are no children by this marriage. There is no family history of diabetes or heart disease. Julius' father died of a CVA at the age of 74 and his mother lived to the age of 92. Presently he is on Medicare. His reason for seeking outpatient care was twitching sensations in his legs.

Physical and Laboratory Findings

Physical examination reveals a Caucasian male, five feet, six inches in height, weight 161 pounds. With the exception of a slight paunch, Julius' manner and bearing is that of a person in his late 50s or early 60s. Blood studies, including cholesterol level, are within normal limits. Suggestions of hyperthyroidism and hypercalcemia were noted. Vision is 20/30 in the right eye and 20/50 in the left eye. Chest X-ray is normal. Blood pressure is 160/80. His heart sounds are normal. Physical examination, including prostate, reveals no abnormalities. In summary, with the exception of possible deranged metabolic status, Julius otherwise appears as a healthy individual for his age status.

Medical Problem Listing

After obtaining the results of all tests, the following problem list was compiled by Julius and his physician.

1. Twitching legs—present for years. No pain accompanies sensation, which diminishes with rigorous rubbing. Julius also notes that with several ounces of Bourbon, the pains also diminish.
2. Enlarging girth—in careful examination of Julius' eating habits, it appears likely that alcoholic intake is primarily responsible.
3. Back trouble—disc surgery was performed seven years ago with good results. Some stiffness develops if strenuous work is undertaken.
4. Formerly a heavy smoker of cigarettes—loose "smoker's cough" present, probably the result of chronic bronchitis.
5. Hyperthyroidism—Julius states that ten years ago a similar condition developed.

Some time after Julius participated in completing the above problem listing, his wife came into the office for a routine checkup. In the course of her visit, she asked if Julius had discussed his recent "blue" period with the doctor. She related that during the past several months, Julius seemed to have lost interest in almost everything. He sits in front of the TV, avoids talking, and appears on the verge of tears much of the time. When questioned by his wife as to what is wrong, Julius withdraws even more and is not communicative.

Based upon this information from his wife, Julius, in a recall visit, was asked about his recent change in behavior. He broke down and told of deep feelings of depression, feelings of unworthiness. In his own words, "I feel like hell and just don't have the spirit to get up and go!" He admitted that he was ashamed to discuss this feeling during the problem-oriented medical workup, and had hoped that some physical cause would be detected to account for these rotten feelings. An appointment was made for Julius to consult with the psychologist.

Personality Profile

The MMPI results obtained by Julius are given in Figure 7–2
    The results suggest that Julius' reality awareness is good. Depression is the outstanding characteristic of the profile. There may be some excessive social sensitivity and some ruminating characteristics, but all in all this appears to be a reactive depression in an essentially normal individual. Individual responses to items suggest concerns about sex and worry concerning "something being wrong with my mind."

Discussion

Julius was seen and asked to describe the "blue spell" he was feeling. He stated that it began three months ago and that he has never had anything like it before in his life. In attempting to relate the onset with outside feelings, Julius said that there was absolutely nothing that was upsetting him three months ago, and in fact, had the "blue spell" occurred two months earlier, he could have understood it. His mother-in-law, to whom Julius was deeply attached, finally died, after being nursed day and night by Julius and his wife. Since the mother-in-law and Julius' wife had always had interpersonal difficulties, Julius' role as nurse and arbitrator was necessary for things to function smoothly. The mother-in-law's death finally occurred at home as she had wished. And after a period of grief, things appeared to return to normal. Julius described in detail the feelings of having "nothing to do" after his mother-in-law's death. He had never enjoyed household activities or gardening and after her death began feeling that nothing

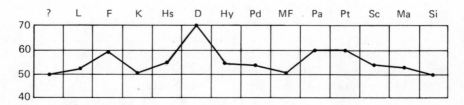

Figure 7–2.

he did had any value or meaning. With this information, the reactive aspects of Julius' depression took on added meaning.

In attempting to shift Julius' perceptions from the past to the present, a discussion followed as to what he would like to be doing at the present time with his life. Julius stated that he would like to go back part-time as a front-end mechanic. He had been away from such work several years, but he expressed confidence that he could do a quality job. He was encouraged to visit some of his old friends in the automobile repair business and to do a "market analysis" of existing opportunities. Another appointment was made for two weeks later.

On the day of the followup appointment, Julius' wife called to say that Julius couldn't keep the appointment. His nephews on the ranch had requested his help and he was down on the ranch helping the nephews brand cattle. His wife was told that this sounded like Julius was out of his "blue" mood, and that if needed, he should contact us upon his return. Six months later Julius had not returned and appeared to be functioning well. He continues to work part-time on the ranch and has apparently achieved a happier outlook concerning his own worth and contributions.

The Case of Martha

Martha, age 52, was referred by a colleague in a small town. She owns her own insurance company, having built it from scratch in five years into a highly successful venture. She has experienced two divorces. The last one occurred five years ago, at which time she began her own business. She has one son, age 30, living in the midwest. She has no allergies, but has been a heavy smoker for 20 years. Previous operations include removal of a benign tumor from the right breast, uterine suspension, appendectomy, hysterectomy, tonsillectomy, two eye surgeries, and the removal of a growth from the bladder, performed cytoscopally. There is no family history of diabetes, rheumatic fever, or TB. Her brother had an aortic graft. Her mother died of a CVA, and a sister had breast cancer. Another brother died of metastatic colon cancer. Her reason for referral was a recurrent abdominal pain in the upper right quadrant. Martha was hospitalized and the problem-oriented process was begun on an inpatient basis.

Physical and Laboratory Findings

Martha is four feet, eleven inches, and weighs 121 pounds. A complete G.I. series including Esophago-Gastro-duodenoscopy was performed. Gastric analysis and duodenal drainage revealed no crystals or inflammatory cells. Blood studies were normal. Chest X-rays revealed no abnormalities, although laboratory findings suggested some limitation of pulmonary function. Liver scan suggested

mild impairment confirmed by liver biopsy. Two upper G.I. series were conducted and both reported negative findings. During the course of her hospital
stay, the patient's depressive tendencies were noted by nursing personnel and
consulting physicians. The possibility of a psychosomatic basis for Martha's
complaints was suggested. While awaiting the results and outcomes of further
diagnostic testing, a problem listing was developed.

Medical Problem Listing

1. Abdominal pain—has been intermittent for years, becoming more persistent
    in the last year. Tends to be associated with emptiness and following in-
    jestion of spicy foods (studies underway).
2. Family history of breast cancer (annual mammogram scheduled).
3. Smoking—heavy smoking and lowered pulmonary function detected.
4. Interpersonal difficulties—two prior divorces, currently living alone with few
    close friends.
5. Bladder tumor—annual urinalisis scheduled.

Because of persistent complaints of pain despite the negative G.I. findings,
the psychological examination was requested on an inpatient basis. A battery of
tests were administered, but only the MMPI results are reported here.

Personality Profile

Martha's MMPI profile and "blind" interpretation is given in Figure 7-3.

Martha's test-taking attitudes appear within normal limits. The mild elevated
F suggests some intellectual disorganization but could be the result of physical
pain. The spike on depression is the outstanding characteristic. Removing the
elevated D scale, elevations on Pd and Ma would suggest a frank, assertive person,
emotional and high strung. With such a profile, there would be suggestions of
social nonconformity or lack of self-control. Her history should be explored to

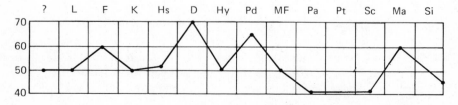

Figure 7-3.

determine if she demonstrates a tendency to get into social scrapes. Alcoholism or the abuse of alcohol is commonly observed in this profile and should be explored in depth. Specific concerns over sexual adjustment and tension level were obtained from her individual answers. Martha indicated that most of the time she wished she was dead. The conclusions drawn from the MMPI:

Patient's responses suggest a reactive depression superimposed upon what might be described as a mild character disorder. It seems likely that for a long period of time Martha has been an outgoing, sometimes norm-violating person who has a tendency to get into difficulties. Marital problems, alcoholism should definitely be explored. The depression observed is probably situationally produced and is of recent origin. Her profile does not suggest hysterical or hypochondrical patterns which would account for her complaints of pain. This is not the sort of personality to complain of vague diffuse pains. Though she might deny over-indulgence on alcohol, this should be explored further.

Discussion

Martha was seen and her feelings of depression discussed. She said that there were many things that were a source of pain to her. Her son has no contact with her, except when he needs financial help. This condition has been chronic for the past five years.

After "botching up" two marriages, Martha decided five years ago to "put a wall around herself" and avoid any involvement with men. She succeeded in accomplishing this until about 12 months ago when she met a client who took her dancing. This man was married to a woman who was supposedly confined to a nursing home with a terminal illness. Martha, over a period of eight months, fell deeply in love with this man. The relationship appeared mutually satisfying until four months ago, when Martha's lover apparently became attracted to a younger woman. Martha attributes her feelings of depression to this. In the meantime, the abdominal pains became more intense.

In conference with the surgeon, the consulting internist, and the psychologist, the decision was made to undertake exploratory surgery despite the negative G.I. findings.

Surgeon's Report

There were some nonserious looking scars over the middle of the liver, suggesting previous trauma. There were many dense adhesions around the gall bladder which did not appear to be grossly abnormal. No stones were seen. The common duct measured about 6/10 of a mm in diameter. There was a huge mass of lymphonodes dorsal to the common duct and around the head of the pancreas. This was quite inflammatory and a section was submitted for pathological study.

The gall bladder was dissected from its bed with sharp and blunt dissection. Care was taken not to encroach upon the relatively narrowed common duct. The choloangiogram was performed midway through the procedure and appeared to be normal. Blood loss was estimated at 100 ccs and the patient returned to the recovery room in good condition.

Following the surgery, with the exception of respiratory difficulties, recovery was uneventful.

Martha was seen on a monthly outpatient basis. She has stopped smoking and is attempting to pace herself in her workload. Her feeling of abandonment by her recent lover is beginning to pass. Considerable improvement in her emotional attitude has been noted since the removal of her gall bladder;

Summary

The three cases reported have attempted to illustrate the pervasiveness of the feelings of depression. Whether Diane's depression is a normal reaction to her sense of loss or a beginning reactive depression, one can only guess. The important contribution that was made in helping Diane was not only to identify the depression, but to interpret her depressive feelings in relation to her other personality characteristics. In this instance, with her shyness and her socially introverted way of life, there appeared a strong possibility that, if left alone, Diane would withdraw further and probably develop even deeper feelings of alienation and loneliness.

Julius represents a delayed reactive depression, a very common normal and/or abnormal phenomenon. Just as important, Julius, age 70, shows some of the attitudes held by older people toward psyche-soma interrelationships. To Julius, an ex-cowboy, rancher and mechanic, the acceptance that grief, a sense of loss, in effect his emotions and feelings, are as important to his well-being as physical needs, some way, somehow seems to denote weakness. One must remember that in Julius' childhood and formative years, the formula for a man to succeed was work hard and keep a stiff upper lip and a tight sphincter!

Martha shows a mild reactive depression of short duration that was probably the result of physical pain as well as her latest interpersonal failure.

Examples such as these are common and routine in almost any primary physician's caseload. Successes with primary reactive depressions treated by brief psychotherapy and the other methods reported here in a general medical setting, have been rapid and successful. Suicide or the threat of suicide is always a major area of concern in dealing with depressive disorders. While this book does not attempt to deal with the area of psychopharmacology, utilization of drugs in the support and treatment of depression is a valuable adjunct. In the observations of the writer, certain mood elevators appear more effective in primary depressive states, while others appear to exacerbate depressive feelings. The indiscriminate prescribing of tranquilizers such as Valium in cases when primary depression is the predominate clinical picture without accompanying complaints of anxiety and psychomotor tension is of questionable value.

References

1. Cross, Harold D. The Problem-Oriented System in Private Practice in a Small Town. *In The Problem-Oriented System.* Baltimore: Williams & Wilkins Co., 1973, p. 159.

2. Kline, N. Practical Management of Depression. *Journal of The American Medical Association* 190(1955):732–40.

3. Westberg, Granger E. *Good Grief.* Philadelphia: Fortress Press, 1962.

4. Beck, Aaron T. *Depression: Clinical, Experimental and Theoretical Aspects.* New York: Harper and Row, 1967, p. 6.

5. Cassidy, W.L.; Flanagan, N.B.; and Spellman, M. Clinical Observations in Manic-Depressive Disease: A Quantitative Study of 100 Manic-Depressive Patients and 50 Medically Sick Controls. *Journal of The American Medical Association* 164(1957):1535–46.

8 Marital Problems in General Medical Practice

In a highly simplified synopsis of the psychological problems facing mankind adopted from Fromm, there appear to be three "acceptances" that a mature individual must ultimately make:[1]

1. acceptance of self,
2. acceptance of others, and
3. acceptance of a philosophy of the meaning of life.

In the acceptance of self, an individual realistically faces his or her deficits and attempts to change or ameliorate such deficits within the limits of his or her ability. In certain types of depression where self-deprecation and self-blame are prominent, the *lack* of self-acceptance is a noticeable symptom. Such terms as "poor self-concept" and "lowered self-esteem" imply a problem in the acceptance of self. Acceptance of others, or the solving of interpersonal problems of self in relation to others—spouses, children, parents, relatives, bosses, competitors—is the subject of this chapter. Malfunctions in acceptance of others are frequently observed in feelings of resentment, suspiciousness, or in some overt psychiatric conditions such as paranoia where the causes of one's difficulties are projected upon others. Finally, in facing the aging process, loneliness, disease, and ultimately death, the need for evolving some religious or philosophical belief system for acceptance of such inevitable consequences of mortality has been postulated. This is not to imply that these three areas of needed acceptance are mutually exclusive. Certainly, one's self-acceptance is greatly influenced by the interpersonal values and feedback one receives from other individuals. A "philosophy of life" stands one in good stead when interpersonal attacks or great personal losses are experienced. The pervasiveness of interpersonal adjustments required in marriage, in divorce, in death of a spouse, in the rearing of children, in coping with the competition and cooperation required to "succeed" in today's economic marketplace makes the acceptance of others one of the most problem-ladened areas in today's long list of necessary adjustments.

As with all institutions, marriage and the family are currently under concerted attack, yet the *number* of families in the United States has increased to

63

47 million and is expected to reach over 55 million by 1980. Altogether some 177 million people, or approximately 92 percent of the population in 1965, lived within some form of family structure.[2] Such data gives tremendous support to the further growth of family practice as a medical necessity.

On the negative side, the rate of divorce is increasing in epidemic proportions. In a recent junior high school visited by the author, over half of the 1,300 children enrolled were either living with a single parent or in a family setting with a stepmother or stepfather. With the many possibilities for the development of interpersonal difficulties that exist, this chapter will focus upon the problem area most frequently encountered in general medical practice—family marital-love relationships.

Increasingly, the emotional and physical disruption of marital discord, separation, and divorce are seen in the patient's listing of problems. Unfortunately, by the time such discord reaches a level where physical symptomotology becomes a part of the picture or the patient can recognize the pain as being generated from this area, it is often too late to effect any substantial change and so the problem becomes one of triage. As Freud observed, love and hate are closely related. The souring of love, the loss of respect toward a loved one, the emptiness that exists when one's most precious gift, the gift of self, is rejected by a loved one create stress only slightly less than that caused by the death of a parent or spouse. The counselor or physician often finds himself in the role of teacher in attempting to help the patient conceptualize the meaning of love.

The word "love" is perhaps the most abused word in the English language. In discussing with patients their difficulties with spouses, children, or sweethearts, persons to whom they profess love, it is revealing and highly diagnostic to ask them their definition of love. Eric Fromm in *The Art of Loving* attempts such a definition.[3] Paraphrasing Fromm, love appears to be the desire to care for, to respect, and to attempt to please another individual. The love relationship, over a period of time, must perform an additional vital function, that of strengthening both the lover and the loved one. To care for someone implies the desire to look after, to provide for the well-being of the other individual. The male image of the husband as the provider for his family or the female image of the mother caring for her children typify this facet. To respect another individual, to allow that person to grow and develop in his *own* image rather than in the image of the lover, is a most difficult and trying aspect of a loving relationship. To attempt to please the loved one by making ones own desires subservient to the wants and desires of the loved one is implied in this portion of the definition. One must hasten to add that such submission of ones own wants and desires must be a *mutual* feeling in which both the lover and the loved one are sensitive to the needs of their mate. The chemistry of the lover and loved one, which over periods of time is actually strengthened by the symbiotic relationship, is a process about which little is known. Unfortunately, the opposite process is more easily demonstrated—a process whereby, with time, the lover and the loved one begin to drain each other, to vent their frustrations upon each other, and to weaken not only the relationship but each other in the process. It is at this stage that help is often requested, but the therapeutic outcome is greatly influenced by the loss of mutual respect that has previously occurred.

Through the romanticized and naive tales of what "true love" should be, there has developed a long list of "family myths" that often are found to be roots of family dissention.[4]

1. Marriage and family should be totally happy, and each individual should of necessity expect (even *demand*) either all or a major part of his or her gratification to come from the family system.
2. Physical proximity, or carrying out most or all activities together—the "togetherness" myth—insures family and individual gratification.
3. Marital partners (or lovers) should be totally honest with one another at all times. Unfortunately, honesty to many persons appears to be primarily negative! (Most "honesty," particularly directed at factors that cannot be changed, is best left unspoken.)
4. A happy marriage is one in which there are no disagreements; and when family members disagree with one another, it means that they hate each other.
5. The marital partners should see eye to eye on all issues and should work toward being as identical in outlook as possible.
6. Marital partners should be as unselfish as possible and give up thinking of their own individual needs.
7. When something goes wrong, one should search to see who is at fault.
8. When things are not going well, it will often be of help to spend a major part of the time analyzing past as well as present hurts.
9. In a marital argument, one partner is "right" and the other is obviously "wrong" and the goal of such arguments is to clearly establish blame.
10. Good sexual relationships will always lead to a good marriage.
11. If the marriage is satisfactory in other respects, the sexual side of it will more or less take care of itself.
12. Marital partners increasingly understand each other's nonverbal communications, so that there is little or no need to check things out with one another verbally.
13. Positive feedback is not as necessary as is negative feedback.
14. A good marriage will "just happen" spontaneously and does not involve any real effort on the part of the participants.
15. Any spouse can (and often *should*) be reformed and remodeled into the shape desired by the partner.
16. A stable marriage is one which things do not change and in which there are no problems.

17. Everyone knows what a husband should be like and what a wife should be like.
18. If a marriage is not working properly, having children will rescue it.
19. No matter how bad the marriage, it should be kept together for the sake of the children.
20. If a marriage does not work, and extramarital affair, or divorce and marriage to another spouse, will cure the situation.

These 20 myths, if studiously adhered to, will insure that married life will be a continuous living hell on earth. Unfortunately, in many dysfunctioning family relationships, certain of these myths form the basis for a marriage union.

One of the most puzzling phenomenas is the breakup of a marriage after 15 or 20 years of fairly stable survival. An interesting and potentially useful theory to account for such events has been developed by Aronson.[5] Through social experimentation, he has demonstrated that the ego-enhancing behavior of a close friend or a loved one over long periods of time comes to be *expected* by the individual. Because we have learned to expect love, favors, and praises from our loved ones, such behaviors do not represent a gain in their esteem for us. By the same token, the loved one has a greater potential to inflict punishment by withholding love, favors, and praise. The closer the person is to us and the greater the past history of that individual's invariant esteem and reward, the more devastating is the withdrawal of love and esteem.

After 20 years of marriage a husband and wife are getting dressed to go out to dinner with friends. The husband compliments her on her appearance. She hears his words, but since he *always* compliments her no matter what she is wearing and thinks she is very attractive, the compliment does not represent a gain in his esteem for her. At the dinner party, a relative stranger engages the wife in conversation and, in apparent sincerity, tells her that she looks positively beautiful. Coming from a stranger, this represents a marked gain in self-esteem for the wife and will not be accepted as matter of fact. While greatly increasing a gain in immediate self-esteem, the stranger runs no risks of becoming a punishment-inflictor by withholding such praise. It appears correct that "you always hurt the one you love." If a relationship is based upon mutual caring and mutual respect, and the relationship has strengthened both the partners over a long period of time, then the inevitable slights and hurts that arise out of sheer proximity do not usually evoke the desire to "hurt back."

If one applies Aronson's tneory to parent-child interactions, then the diminishing ego-enhancing gains that the parents are able to transmit to the child through praise, love, and concern would provide some insight into the crises between parents and teenagers. At the adolescent stage, the parents' ego-enhancement may add little to the teenager's self-esteem. The withdrawal of such parental praise, love, and concern, however, may have a tremendously disrupting effect upon the teenager's feelings of gain in self-esteem. This apparent contradiction is one of the severe occupational hazards of parenthood which normally solves itself through the increased growth and maturity of the child. In some instances, however, the role of Mama and Papa remains fixated at the adolescent ambivalent level, capable only of reassuring the child in times of stress and having little, if any, positive ego-enhancing growth effects. Whether such a state of affairs is a deficit in the parent, the child, or both requires intensive investigation.

It seems highly significant in reviewing the case load of the past three years that all medical patients who indicate marital distress, and who further indicate desire for help within this area, have been women. Men apparently do not want to perceive the pain and discomfort of a malfunctioning marriage within the total context of health. Using a problem-oriented medical approach with male patients seldom results in the incorporation of family problems into the finalized protocol. When such family or marital problems do exist, the *symptoms* of discomfort are more often noted by male medical patients. Problems such as "insomnia," "feelings of anxiety or tension," or "depression," listed as major health problems in a married male patient, require considerable investigation to determine the quality of interpersonal relationships which exist between the patient and his wife, his children, or other individuals to whom he professes love. Interpersonal tensions on the job and the resulting discomfort and distress produced are readily advanced by males as contributing to health problems. Taken in total context, it is likely that the male patients' reluctance to include marital-family interpersonal problems as health concerns, while freely discussing job stresses or difficulties with superiors or employees, is a form of macho or false male ego. Bartenders probably provide the bulk of psychotherapy in such cases!

Attempting to help a patient, usually a female, with a family-marital problem in a general medical setting is approached in the same way as with any other behavioral/emotional condition. If the patient includes such problems as significant in her total health protocol and indicates a desire for help, treatment plans are developed, psychodiagnostic procedures are undertaken, and the findings are integrated into the total medical workup. Attempting to counsel with an individual experiencing a marital problem differs from one-to-one therapy in several ways. After initial assessment of the patient's current functioning status, which is often colored greatly by the stress of separation, marital discord, or divorce, some prognosis for the possibility of reconciliation between the patient and the spouse must be made. If the love erosion has not gone past the point of no return, the early stages of individual therapy/counseling are usually spent in trying to determine if, for the patient's future emotional happiness, an effort at reconciliation should be made. Unfortunately, in over half the cases treated, divorce proceedings had been initiated or divorce had already occurred.

If reconciliation appears as a possibility and the patient wishes to "try again," a second level of decisions must be faced. If family counseling or psychotherapy with the spouse appears necessary, who should undertake this effort? Should the same therapist see both the husband and the wife? Should conjoint counseling be attempted? Such questions can only be determined on a case-by-case basis. In any event, *any* contact between the therapist and the spouse of a patient occurs only with the complete support and acceptance of the patient. In the case material presented, discussions of such decisions, which are required at the various stages of marital counseling/psychotherapy, are included.

The Case of Lucille

Lucille is a 34-year-old full-time housewife. She is a high school graduate who has been employed as a teacher's aide during the past year. She is married to a supervisor in a manufacturing establishment and there is a 14-year-old son from this union. She currently is serving as a part-time secretary in a local church. She sought medical help from rectal bleeding—suspected hemorrhoids. There is a family history of breast cancer and colon cancer. Her husband is recovering from five-stage urethroplasty. The patient had total hysterectomy four years ago.

Physical and Laboratory Workup

The patient is attractive but overweight: weight 148 pounds, height five feet, seven inches. Through dieting she has lost over 20 pounds in the past six months. Her blood pressure was 110/80. Blood studies revealed slightly lowered red blood count. Urinalysis was normal. Sigmoidoscopy revealed rectal surface hemorrhoids. Breast examination revealed tenderness in right breast and mammogram results were inconclusive. Biopsy was performed. Pelvic examination was negative.

Medical Problem Profile

Following the results of the physical and laboratory workup, the following problem list was developed between the patient and the general physician.

1. Hemorrhoids—minor in nature and will likely respond to injection. No surgery required at present.
2. Epigastric burning pains—upper G.I. series revealed no gross pathology.
3. Urinary distress—occasional incontinence. Becomes much more prominent with stress.
4. Tenderness in right breast—biopsy negative. With strong history of breast cancer, mammograms will be scheduled on a yearly basis.

5. Marital problems—almost no communication between patient and husband. Counseling with minister during past two years.

Approximately two months after the problem-oriented medical workup, Lucille called the office in an extremely agitated state, reporting that her husband had packed his belongings and told her he was seeking a divorce. She told of her feelings of depression and hoplessness and voiced a concern that she might attempt to take her own life as she had once attempted some ten years ago. An appointment was immediately scheduled for Lucille to come to the office. An hour was spent with the patient, who alternated between tearfulness and rage. An appointment was scheduled for the following day for psychodiagnosis.

Personality Profile

On the MMPI, the profile shown in Figure 8–1 was obtained.

The results suggest some slippage in reality awareness and very low ego strength. Individuals with similar profiles frequently complain of agitated depression with accompanying tension, self-doubts and insecurity, and "nervousness." These problems are likely of long standing but undoubtedly are elevated by the current stress of marital separation. Answers to specific items reveal dissatisfaction with sex life, and a suggestion that on occasion the patient feels like harming herself or others. With a past history of a suicide attempt and the heightened depression and tension level, there was concern that this patient would not be able to cope and might require hospitalization. Alternative hospitalization plans were prepared in the event outpatient treatment could not obtain fairly immediate results.

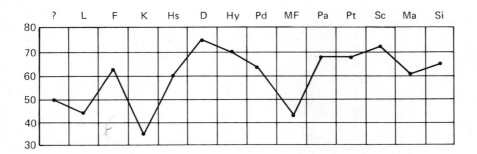

Figure 8–1.

Discussion

Lucille was seen twice a week for a total of six sessions. In the course of these sessions, the following additional history material emerged. Lucille was the only child in an Italian family. Against her family wishes, she met and married her huband outside of the Roman Catholic Church at age 18. She moved to Nevada with him to an army base after marriage. Being alone and homesick, she returned to her family after six months. Her failure to remain with her husband was frequently thrown at her by her family, particularly her mother and aunts. Her father supported her emotionally during this trying period, until her husband was discharged from the service. Sexual problems between her and her husband developed upon his return from the service. Frequency of intercourse at age 20 was twice per month and steadily diminished. The husband sought medical care where prostatic difficulties were discovered and corrected by surgery. Sex and sex problems have always been a source of concern and feelings of inferiority to both the patient and, in her eyes, to her husband. A son was conceived and delivered when the patient was 20 years old and the closeness between son and mother since his birth is very apparent, with the mother and son frequently on one side of arguments and the husband on the other. For the past 14 years the psychological distance between the patient and her husband has been increasing. The one admitted attempt at suicide occurred seven years ago. While preparing to attend a wedding, the patient, much overweight at the time, was attempting to dress for the affair. Her husband, impatient because they were to be in the wedding part and appeared to be late, made some cutting remark to the patient. Lucille locked herself in the bathroom and swallowed 15 sleeping pills. In describing the incident, she said it was a sudden, impulsive thing: "Why put up with this pain? I don't want to live."

During these six sessions the patient's mood swung widely from hostility and rage directed toward her husband and a recounting of all the selfish acts that he had ever performed, to self-pity and fear that she could not cope alone. Aided by medication, her wide mood swings began to abate. Two weeks after the initial separation, she received the divorce papers, which upset her temporarily. In order to keep herself occupied, she was encouraged to return to her prior job as teacher's aide when the opportunity was given her. Weekly contacts were maintained for two months because of her job schedule.

After the initial rage reaction coupled with self-pity receded, the possibility of reconciliation was never discussed. The divorce was finalized with a minimum of bitterness. The patient has continued to keep her weight down in the year since the divorce and occasionally dates, with no serious emotional involvements up to the present. The son is now 16 years old, and a student leader and an A student in high school. The boy's graduation from high school and possible college attendance will likely be a difficult stage of growth for Lucille. If further support and help are needed, hopefully Lucille will return. In the meantime, she continues to come in periodically for physical checkups and preventive tests in connection with her other health problems. Lucille's case could just as easily had been included in a chapter entitled crisis intervention rather than in a chapter dealing with interpersonal/marital problems.

The Case of Louanne

This 30-year-old housewife lives on a ranch in an outlying small town with her husband and two sons, ages nine and five. She currently serves on a national rodeo committee and her hobbies are centered around horses, riding, and horse breeding. There is no family history of rheumatic fever, breast cancer, or diabetes. The major reason for seeking help is her "nerves."

Physical and Laboratory Workup

The patient is five feet, four inches, and weighs 125 pounds. Blood and urinalysis are negative. The patient wears contact lenses for myopia. Breast and pelvic examinations reveal no abnormalities, with the exception of vaginitis which the patient has experienced in the last eight months. Pap test was normal; vaginitis appeared as result of infection, confirmed by smear test.

Medical Problem Profile

In collaboration with Louanne, the following medical problems were identified and rank ordered.

1. Vaginitis—treatment by topical antibiotics.
2. Weight gain of ten pounds in the past six months—appeared to be high fat an sugar intake related.
3. Increasing marital disharmony for past 18 months.—
4. Smoking—a lifetime habit which has increased to two packs per day in the last year.

Dietary counseling was given concerning the weight gain. As to the increased marital tension, the patient indicated that she would like to talk with someone about this problem. Both she and her husband had gone to a marriage counselor for two sessions, but have not continued. Louanne was scheduled to see the psychologist.

Personality Profile

On the MMPI, Louanne obtained the results given in Figure 8-2.

The results suggest that Louanne took the MMPI in good faith, neither over- or underexaggerating her responses. Elevated K suggests high ego strength and possibly some emotional defensiveness. Elevated Ma suggests an enterprising, energetic individual who under stress might be expected to attempt to cope with anxiety by doing things rather than internalizing such anxiety. She appears to be socially extroverted and gains satisfaction from people-related activities.

Discussion

In discussing Louanne's marriage, she told of meeting her husband while in high school, and his being two years older. He was the youngest son of three, born to an immigrant family who acquired a large area of land and, through hard work, became highly successful and wealthy ranchers. Because of her different ethnic background the patient has never been accepted by her husband's family. Her huband has become very suspicious of her activities with the rodeo association. He is highly critical of her housekeeping abilities and, in the patient's view, appears to be looking for things to criticize about her actions and her thoughts. For the past two years, Louanne has kept more and more of her thoughts to herself. Sexual contacts are less and less frequent. Louanne spends more and more of her time with her horses, and in social activities outside the home—bridge playing, school PTA activities, horse breeding. A trial separation of three weeks occurred six months previously but ended with her husband returning home, asking forgiveness, and promising to not be so critical of his wife's behavior. Louanne's smoking is a particularly obnoxious habit to her husband. He has asked her repeatedly to quit, and appears to interpret her continuing to smoke as a defiance of his authority. From viewing the patient's MMPI and from the impressions obtained in two interviews, it appeared as though Louanne's husband might be more in need of help than Louanne. Louanne readily agreed with

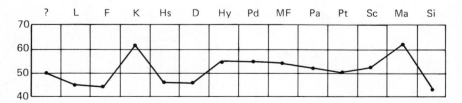

Figure 8–2.

this and asked if the therapist would see her husband. After discussing with the patient the pitfalls in this approach, the therapist agreed that if the husband was willing, he would be seen. A telephone call from the husband two days later established his concern and willingness for help. Prior to seeing Louanne's husband, he completed the MMPI with the following results.

Husband's Responses

As indicated by Figure 8–3, Louanne's husband appears to be exhibiting some looseness in his thinking. His ego strength appears at a very low ebb. The peaks and degree of elevation suggest rather severe depression, along with considerable sensitivity and hostility, and weak impulse control. Individuals with similar profiles are described as shy, sensitive, prone to worry, self-dissatisfied but exhibiting strong hostility, resentment, and impulsiveness, usually of a long-standing nature.

These results substantiate the original hypothesis that Louanne's husband is exhibiting more symptoms of pathology than his wife, and probably is experiencing much more difficulty in coping with the marital discord than she is. In responding to individual items Louanne's husband suggests problems in impulse control, in hurting himself and others, a constant feeling of tension and anxiety, and concern over sexual problems.

Interviews with Louanne's Husband

Louanne's husband immediately launched into a scathing attack of his wife's coldness, her selfishness, and her actions, which the husband interprets as being calculated to upset him. Her smoking was an obsession with him, and he stated, "If she loved me enough, she would be willing to stop doing those things which upset me." It became clear that, to Louanne's husband, human behavior was

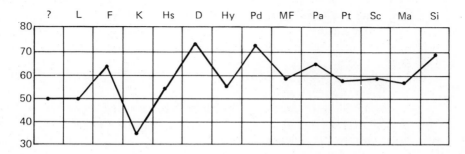

Figure 8–3.

purely animalistic, i.e.: a system of reward and punishment. Any realization that love implied respect for the right of the loved one to behave in a different manner could not be tolerated by this man. Both of his brothers had experienced divorces and/or separations in the past year, and his regard of a wife as a property item appeared to be very deep-seated. His jealousy and intolerance of his wife's hobbies, her social activities, and particularly her rodeo activities, which put her in contact with other men, were also deeply resented.

When asked about prior efforts at marital counseling, Louanne's husband said it was so much "bull shit," because the marriage counselor "beat around the bush" and talked in such a low, quiet voice that he could not understand him. (The husband complained of a hearing problem which was service-related. This was later confirmed.) After two sessions with Louanne's husband, it became apparent that insight-oriented nondirective therapy would be of no benefit. A judgment was made to "lay it on the line" to the husband and interpret to him the inconsistencies of his attitudes and behavior toward the usual norms of love—to care for, respect, please, and strengthen and be strengthened by a love relationship.

In a conjoint meeting with Louanne and her husband, the severity and poor prognosis for the ultimate patching up of their floundering marriage was discussed with both participants. The alternative suggested was that they return to their marriage counselor and attempt to work through their differences, accepting the fact that the process would be long range and would require a tremendous commitment and willingness to change on both their parts. If such a commitment could not be mutually acceptable, then dissolving the marriage without further hurt and pain should be considered.

Louanne and her husband apparently decided to return to the marriage counselor in their own community, for a release for information signed by both Louanne and her husband was received two weeks later. In subsequent followup, it has been learned that Louanne and her husband are now legally separated, with a divorce pending. Louanne has obtained employment in the small town bank as an apprentice teller, and appears to be weathering the separation and divorce. The husband has returned to the family home, where he and his brothers are apparently offering each other support in their divorce actions and marital failures.

The Case of Madeline

This 24-year-old, full-time housewife was born in a rural area and married at age 17 to a man two years her senior. There are two children, a boy age eight and a girl age six. The boy has epilepsy, Grand mal, which appears to be controlled by Dilatin. Since diagnosis two years ago, the frequency of seizures has diminished, with only rare episodes. There is no history of cariovascular disease, diabetes, breast cancer, or rheumatic fever. Hobbies include all forms of outdoor activities, and sewing, homemaking, and creative decorating. Her principal reason for seeking medical help was "progressive fatigue and tiredness" during the past six months.

Physical and Laboratory Workup

The patient is five feet, seven and one-half inches, and weighs 130 pounds. Her blood pressure is 110/70. Blood studies reveal lowered red blood cell count and iron deficiency. Pelvic examination revealed a cervititis, which appeared to be chronic. Pap smear test was negative. Patient evidenced some feeling of tenderness in the uterine area. Breast examination revealed no abnormalities.

Medical Problem Profile

Upon completion of the physical and laboratory studies, the following problem list was developed with the patient.

1. Interpersonal difficulties with husband—Such stress periods have been experienced for the past four years. Marital counseling was received five years ago with improvement noted.
2. Chronic cervititis—Has been a recurrent condition during the past three years. She has been treated by antibiotics and electrical cauterization. D&C discussed with the patient and plans made for procedure to be conducted within the next month. Referral to obstetrician-gynecologist consultant also discussed.
3. Heavy smoking of cigarettes—In excess of two packs per day.

In discussing problem 1, the patient indicated that she would like to obtain help with her marital problems and an appointment was made with the psychologist.

Personality Profile

On the MMPI, the patient obtained the profile shown in Figure 8–4.
Patient's attitude toward testing suggests some defensiveness, which could be interpreted as ego strength. While within normal limits, patient's peak of Pd suggests some difficulty with impulse control. Reactions to stress might be to react impulsively with minor depressive and somatic reactions.

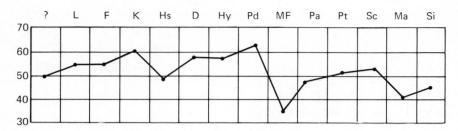

Figure 8–4.

Discussion

Three one-hour sessions were spent with Madeline discussing her interpersonal problems with her husband. Her marriage was opposed by her parents because of her age (16) and the immaturity of both herself and her husband-to-be. Her husband raced stock cars, and during the first year of marriage spent three months away from his pregnant wife, while touring the stock car racing circuit. Upon his return home he was cold to his wife, and indicated that he had met other women to whom he was attracted. With considerable pressure from both families, the young couple remained together. The husband made economic ends meet by working as a ranch hand, and with some financial help from parents. Approximately three years ago the young couple left their rural home town and moved to a large city suburb, where the husband was engaged in landscaping. Economically, the husband made a good living in this activity until he was laid off. Madeline obtained a three-quarter-time job and worked for a year while her husband was unemployed. Lack of concern on her husband's part, and his lack of motivation in seeking employment, apparently created marital tensions and led to marital counseling three years ago. Since then, the husband has been working steady.

Some three weeks ago, after attending a party and drinking quite heavily, the husband proposed that he and his wife should experiment with "wife swapping." Apparently he had discussed this with another male acquaintance. This proposition upset Madeline tremendously, and brought out many of the ambivalent feelings that she had harbored toward her husband since their marriage. During the course of discussion, she expressed considerable insight as to the type of man she had married. He has continually been an "experimentor" in many areas. He smoked pot quite regularly until Madeline "put her foot down." He is inclined to be irresponsible in financial obligations unless kept on track by the patient. In many ways, Madeline functions as the mother of the entire family, including her husband.

After three sessions, the patient was asked if she felt that she would be able to rekindle her feelings toward her husband. She deliberated and finally, in a resigned manner, stated that this appeared to be a repetition of previous cycles. His irresponsibility created hostility within her. After a period of about a month, her hostilities abated, and she once more assumed her prior role as planner and mother. When asked if intervention with the husband might help, she replied that she did not know, but agreed to discuss this with her husband. Two weeks later she called the therapist to say that she felt she had her feelings back in perspective, and indicated that her husband would like at least to meet with the therapist and that she would appreciate the therapist doing what he could to increase her husband's understanding of the marital differences.

Discussion with Husband

In discussing the precipitating factor that had upset Madeline, the husband reacted rather sheepishly. When discussing their prior marital problems, he admitted his immaturity and impulsive nature. He indicated that he was trying, but spoke of his wife's "coldness" and unforgiving manner after one of his indiscretions. The husband's immaturity and dependence on Madeline was very evident. He was not willing to enter into a therapeutic relationship to attempt to understand himself better. Therefore, no MMPI results could be obtained. The prognosis for Madeline's marriage appears poor, based upon the lack of maturity on the part of her husband and his apparent unwillingness to face her needs squarely. While the marriage is still intact, it is likely that, within the next several years, the "cycle," as Madeline calls it, will recur and a qualitative change will occur in this tenuous relationship.

Summary

The cases included in this chapter may appear rather pessimistic because of the outcomes. In the case of Lucille, therapy was directed at maintaining her own equilibrium in the face of the crisis of separation and divorce. With Louanne and her husband, efforts at marital counseling also had a flavor of crisis intervention, rather than of constructive therapy per se. In the case of Madeline, until more motivation is observed on the part of her husband, little that is constructive can be accomplished.

Such results are really no different from those obtained in mental health centers. If the goal of marital counseling is reconciliation, then a 15 percent "cure rate" appears realistic. If, on the other hand, one views marital problems as forms of crisis, then the goal of such therapy shifts to support of the patient through such a crisis with minimal personality damage. In general medical settings, this latter view appears the more pragmatic because of the stage of disintegration that most marriage problems evidence by the time they reach the primary medical practitioner's attention. Perhaps as family medical practice becomes more accepted, problems in marital and family interpersonal relations can be detected at a much earlier stage and more fruitful intervention and educational methods devised to prevent the emotional and behavioral problems that such disruptions produce in the health of general medical patients.

References

1. Fromm, Erick. *Escape from Freedom*. New York: Farrar and Rinehart, 1941.

2. Glick, Ira D., and Kessler, David R. *Marital and Family Therapy*. New York: Grune and Stratten, 1974, pp. 1-2.

3. Fromm, Erick. *The Art of Loving*. New York: Harper & Row, 1956.

4. Glick and Kessler, *Marital and Family Therapy*.

5. Aronson, Elliot. *The Social Animal*. San Francisco: W.H. Freeman, 1972, pp. 224-33.

9 Psychoneuroses in General Medical Practice

The term psychoneuroses, by implication and definition, conveys a labeling of a "functional" disorder of feelings and emotions of an individual to some real or anticipated stress or conflict. Bodily reactions to organic diseases are also "functionally determined" reactions of stress to the organism. The differentiation between a neurotic reaction and an organic reaction is exceedingly difficult to make, and requires the best collaborative thinking of both the physician and the psychologist. Even with such collaborative diagnostic efforts, in almost half the cases the conclusion is one of *both* psychoneurotic *and* organic causative factors. Neuroses, through the autonomic nervous system, may actually produce organic disease. Organically caused illnesses may create an overlay of psychoneurotic symptoms.

The labeling of a general medical patient as neurotic, based solely upon negative results from the physical and laboratory workup, appears to be a hazardous procedure for the primary medical practitioner. It is suspected that such diagnoses by general physicians form the basis for a good number of ultimate malpractice suits. Conversely, the mental health worker who, after obtaining supposedly clear evidence that a psychoneurotic condition exists in a patient, does not insure that physical conditions which may be influencing such a "neurotic" reaction are identified and corrected, also opens himself to claims of malpractice. The following experience taught the writer a very meaningful lesson.

While visiting in a physician friend's office on a personal matter, the writer was asked to see one of his patients for a short consultation. It seems that this 68-year-old married woman had been suffering a vague pain in the abdominal area for the past month. Prior surgery included gall bladder removal and a hysterectomy seven years before. During the past month the patient had received two upper G.I. series and glucose tolerance tests with negative results. A consultation with a cardiologist had been obtained with negative findings. In discussing this with the patient, she told of her efforts to determine the cause of discomfort. "I swallowed all that chalk solution twice. All I heard was that the tests were all normal. Then I went to this doctor and he took a cardiogram. He kept

79

looking at the records, never looking at me or asking about *my* pain, and he kept saying 'There's nothing wrong with your heart'."

When asked to describe the pain, the woman said it usually had an onset between midnight and 1:00 A.M. after she had been asleep for two hours or more. It was like a severe heartburn, and usually receded in 30 minutes after ingestion of soda or gelusil. It was suggested that she place a pencil and paper by her bedside and when awakened, note the time the pain awakened her. (This she did for a week, and on the four nights in which she experienced discomfort, the pains occurred between 12:30 and 1:30 A.M.) The patient was a frail, underweight person whose husband, a plumber, liked his dinner promptly at 5:00 P.M. After watching the TV until 9:00 P.M., the patient and her husband went to bed, always by 10:00 P.M. In consultation with the physician, the possibility of digestive causes were discussed. The patient was encouraged to eat a piece of pie or cake with a big glass of milk prior to retiring, and to continue to keep a log of her awakenings with the pain. Since starting this regime, she has not experienced the pain.

Taking this example to its extreme, the "cause" of the woman's discomfort was not known. Blood studies, glucose tolerance tests, G.I. series, and cardiograms showed no findings that would account for her pain. By relying only upon test findings, it might be tempting to draw the following logical conclusion: "The tests for possible potential causes of this pain have been eliminated; therefore, it must be emotional (mental, psychosomatic, neurotic, etc.)." Such a conclusion might have led to a recommendation to the patient to seek help from a mental health worker. (Listening intently to the patient's description of her condition, without preconceived hypotheses as to causality, is another lesson that this example illustrates.) Suppose, further, that the patient did seek psychological diagnosis and treatment, and that in the course of history taking, the possible physical relationship between the patient's pain and duration of time since eating dinner was noted, and brought to the physician's attention as the possible cause. Defensiveness of the part of the physician could occur when his patient was referred back to him, after psychological diagnoses, suggesting that physical causal factors be further explored. This type of interaction in both the diagnostic and treatment stages may occur many times if the patient's condition does not respond to treatment.

For the physician to discover hypoglycemia or thyroid malfunctioning in a patient with all the symptoms and behavior of a psychoneurotic, and to observe the patient's so-called functional emotional symptoms abate, is a humbling experience to the psychologist. Such experiences are common when true collaboration between physician and psychologist exists. When such instances occur, particularly in the area of diagnosis and treatment of suspected psychoneurosis, the gains to the patient far outweigh the ego deflation that might occur for the healers.

Psychoneuroses are characterized by the intact reasoning and conceptualization of the sufferer. There is no failure to perceive the external environment realistically. On the average, the sufferer of a neurosis is usually above average intellectually. Instead, the neurosis sufferer is literally "his own worst enemy." His complaints may be "nerves," anxiety, fearfulness of real or anticipated stresses, feelings of inadequacy, depression, self-doubt, physiological reactions directly attributable to his sympathetic nervous system, or even bizarre rituals devised by the patient to ward off his inner anxieties or fears. The chief factor to keep in mind when dealing with someone suffering from a neurosis (note the avoidance of the terms "psychoneurotic" or "neurotic"), is that the patient is actually in pain. In case material presented in earlier chapters, particularly for Gene in Chapter 6, it can be observed that many sufferers of neuroses actually welcome a physical disability that gives them an acceptable medical reason for feeling as badly as they do.

Another reaction to the sufferer of a neurosis by some physicians is to "give the patient hell" for his vague complaints, unreasonable fears, and "silly" emotions. Usually such a reaction only produces one of two results—the patient no longer verbalizes his feelings to the physician, or the patient moves on to another physician. "Doctor shopping" is common occurrence among sufferers of neuroses. A preliminary listing of characteristics of the psychoneurosis may be helpful at this point.

Clinical Criteria for the Diagnosis of Neuroses[1]

1. *The presence of anxiety.* The presence of disruptive anxiety is observed in certain stages of almost all forms of psychoneurosis. The anxiety may be continuous or episodic in nature, involving not only the exaggerated worries or fears within the emotions of the sufferer, but also including bodily functions as concomitants of that anxiety. To elicit carefully the subject of the fears, and to explore fully the conflict, the situation, or the conditions around which the patient experiences anxiety, and the onset and duration of such anxiety feelings, is a critical activity that must be very carefully undertaken before conclusions are made as to the presence of a neurosis. Within the health protocols of problems in general medical settings, the inclusion of anxiety, tension or "nerves" as a major health problem is very common.

2. *The presence of irrational thoughts or overt behaviors by which the patient attempts to contain or control anxieties, worries and/or fears.* Obsessions, repetitive thoughts that appear outside the control of the patient, compulsive acts, and phobic reactions to certain situations, conditions, or circumstances fall into this category. Classical examples of obsessive-compulsive psychoneurosis are relatively rare in health problems presented by general medical patients. In instances where such complaints are encountered, a previous history of psychiatric or psychological help is usually encountered.

3. *The presence of sensorimotor or psychosomatic dysfunctions that cannot be totally accounted for by organic findings.* Again, "pure" hysterical neuroses have been observed only in isolated instances and usually following surgery. The complaint of excruciating pain following minor surgery or the inability to move a part of the body following a minor trauma may contain some elements of conversion hysteria neurosis, but such occurrences as "stocking anesthesia," hysterical blindness, and total paralysis of a limb are rare. Psychosomatic complaints (or somatopsychic complaints), on the other hand, are very common. Dizziness, flushing, insomnia, sensations of hot or cold flashes, respiratory problems, skeletal muscular aches and pains, together with gastrointestinal and digestive disorders, are frequently reported with the emotional feelings and/or sensations. Since such sensations are also bona fide symptoms of a wide range of organic disorders, to merely use a "wastebasket" diagnosis of neurosis after a preliminary medical workup on patients presenting such complaints is very risky.

4. *The shifting of complaints from one organ system to another.* Over a period of time and with repeated contacts, the physician may note a shifting of complaints from headaches, to dermatitis, to G.I. complaints, to complaints of weakness and fatigue. The ubiquitousness of the complaints over periods of time gives some clues as to psychogenic origin.

5. *The onset of symptoms under circumstances of conflict or emotional stress.* To elicit from the patient a chronological sequence of the stresses to which he has been subjected, and then to determine if the symptom complaints appear correlated with such occurrences, is a diagnostic procedure that aids in determining if the symptoms may be socially, emotionally, or environmentally produced. Some individuals, when faced with a crisis, may become very agitated and upset *prior* to the actual crisis and then settle down and wade through the situation with no outward signs of discomfort. Others may confront the crisis, apparently weather the discomfort, and then, three to six months later, "let down" and demonstrate a delayed reaction. When attempting to apply this criteria to determine if the particular behavior or complaint has a psychogenic element, it is well to remember that individual reactions to stress are highly individualistic, and are not purely mechanical or neurological responses.

6. *The "secondary gain" that the symptom or complaint provides in protecting the sufferer from uncomfortable or stress-producing situations.* According to Freud's "Pleasure-Pain Theory," if a particular behavior, no matter how uncomfortable or bizarre, actually protects the sufferer from far more uncomfortable situations or conflicts, then there is little motivation for change.[2] A woman complains of periodic urine retention problems and needs surgical attention to correct this incontinence. If she is socially introverted and her condition actually gives her a socially acceptable excuse to remain at home and avoid such feared social contacts, the prognosis for getting patient acceptance for corrective procedures is poor.

These six criteria are at best "rules of thumb" that can be applied in attempting to formalize a diagnosis of psychoneurosis. All six imply that a longitudinal study of the patient by the physician occurs over time. The additional information supplied from psychological instruments such as the MMPI supplements the physician's observations and adds an additional dimension to this judgmental process. Anxiety reactions and depressive reactions of a psychoneurotic nature comprise the great majority of emotional/behavioral problems encountered in general medical practice. Perhaps because of the medical setting, such anxiety and depressive reactions are usually accompanied by specific somatic complaints. Even brief counseling sessions (from one to three contacts), providing the patient with insight and knowledge as to how his or her feelings and emotions actually produce physiological changes, seem to materially lower the added apprehension and anxiety that the fear of organic difficulties brings. While such a procedure does little to cure the subjective pain experienced by the sufferer of a neurosis, it at least points him in the direction of the source of his physical and emotional discomfort.

The Case of Mary

Mary, a 52-year-old full-time housewife, was referred by her family physician because of recurrent cramps and urinary incontinence. Up until two years ago, the patient worked part-time as a grocery store checker and in the lunchroom of a neighborhood school, but because of increased physical discomfort, she stopped such outside activities.

Mary's prior operations include hysterectomy at age 45, an appendectomy at age 34, and a varicose vein operation at age 50. She received treatment for gastric ulcer during the past five years, and has suffered numerous bladder infections. She feels "blue" at the prospects of further physical troubles requiring surgery. For the past six months, she has withdrawn from social contacts, and has received less enjoyment from hobbies such as needlepoint, knitting, and baking. Family history reveals no diabetes or heart disease. There is a history of cancer on the maternal side of Mary's family. Her mother died of cancer at age 64. Her father died at age 81 of old age. Patient reports long history of anemia.

Physical and Laboratory Workup

The patient is five feet, six inches, weighs 140 pounds. Blood pressure was recorded as 130/80. Urinalysis revealed no abnormalities. Blood studies revealed lower estrogen, hypothyroidism, and red count. Tenderness noted in lower left quadrant of abdomen. Barium enema ordered to compare with previous berium enemas in 1974 and 1975. Sigmoidoscopic examination revealed no abnormalities for 20 cm. Results of berium enema revealed diverticular disease. In con-

sultation with the surgeon, a two stage Sigmoid resection for diverticular disease
was recommended.

Medical Problem Profile

Upon completion of the physical and with the results of the laboratory tests,
the following listing of problems was developed by Mary and the physician:

1. Diverticular disease—Three specific attacks have occurred in the past two
   years. Surgery required.
2. Urinary incontinence—occurs daily with coughing and lifting. Occurs less
   frequently with estrogen intake. Patient is very sensitive concerning this, and
   avoids social situations because of it. If problem 1 is surgically undertaken,
   perhaps this problem could also be corrected.
3. Low back pain—Three cortisone shots have been administered in lumbar
   spine in past year. Patient shows full range of motion. Possibly related to
   diverticular disease. To reassess after surgery.
4. Hypothyroidism—Has been on medication for years, clinically appears ec-
   thyroid. Will take off medicine and evaluate thyroid functioning, which
   could be contributing to lifelong problem of anemia.
5. Smoking—Has consumed a pack a day for many years. No coughing and
   arterial blood gases appear normal. This condition must be kept in mind
   postoperatively.
6. Attitude of depression—Gets "blue" when she looks back on her many
   physical difficulties and the prospects of another two-stage operation.
7. History of gastric ulcer—While not a factor at this time, this should be kept
   in mind both pre- and postoperatively.

Three weeks after initial workup, the patient underwent an uneventful sub-
total colectomy. Biopsy of excised tissue was negative. The patient recovered
uneventfully and returned home after ten days, fully capable of changing the
temporary colostomy container. Six weeks later, the final surgical step was
completed, closing the colostomy, and the patient gained control of normal
bowel movements. She has been seen on an outpatient basis for four weeks
following final surgery. Physical healing progressed nicely; however, her depression and social isolation tendencies continue. At this point, she was referred
for psychodiagnostic appraisal and possible counseling.

Personality Profile

On the MMPI, Mary obtained the results given in Figure 9-1:
   Mary's attitude toward taking the test appears open, with little defensiveness

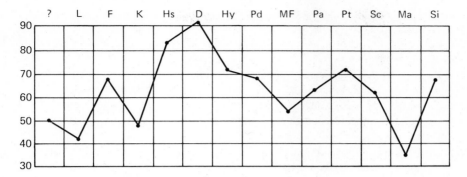

Figure 9–1

or self-protection. The elevated F suggests some "looseness" in thinking. The severe elevations on depression and hypochondriasis suggest an individual who complains of feeling emotionally "bottled up." Individuals with similar elevations frequently express feelings of self-doubt, insecurities, and lack of interest or involvement in activities, along with complaints of fatigue and nervousness. In general, marked periods of anxiety or tension are infrequent. Instead, the complaints are of long standing, suggesting that such patients have a high tolerance for unhappiness. Frequent marital problems are reported among patients with similar profiles, but divorce is rare. A diagnosis of psychoneurosis with depression and hypochondriacal concerns appears warranted.

Discussion

Mary has recovered nicely from the two-stage diverticular corrective surgery. She now is apprehensive concerning whether or not surgery will be required for her bladder incontinence problem. In the initial interview, Mary attempted to keep the discussion on a strictly physically oriented level, relating her past and present surgeries. When the MMPI results were interpreted to her, she heaved a sigh of relief and told of her lifelong difficulties in expressing her true feelings without fear of reprisal. She related a childhood marred by continuous friction with her mother, who, in the patient's mind, was constantly nagging, picking at details, and tearing the patient down. The oldest of three children, she eloped at the age of 17 and married a truck driver, for which her mother never forgave her. This marriage was unhappy from the very beginning. Mary's husband drank excessively and was exceedingly controlling and possessive. In order to make ends meet, Mary was forced to take part-time jobs as a waitress and as a receptionist. Four children were produced from this first marriage. Infidelities, economic crises, and constant friction were continuous occurrences.

After 17 years of marriage, Mary's first husband was killed in a truck-automobile accident, leaving Mary totally responsible for the economic welfare of the four children. While working at two jobs, one as a part-time bartender in a service club, she met her present husband. In her own words, "He was different in every way from my first husband. He was considerate, gentle, and, most importantly, I felt he would be good for the kids". This union now is in its seventeenth year. Ten years ago, following surgery for prostate removal, her husband became totally impotent. Only within the last year, along with her diverticular problems, has Mary begun feeling ambivalent toward her present husband. His placidness, once a highly regarded attribute, now gets on the patient's nerves. When this occurs, Mary's guilt and depression increase because of her gratefulness to her present husband over his acceptance and continued support of the children.

Gentle encouragement was given Mary to attempt to begin to share some of her feelings with her husband. Her willingness to discuss with her husband possible medical and/or psychological help for his impotency was broached. Mary promised to take such suggestions under advisement and when the appropriate time occurred, to attempt to discuss such topics with her husband. As to her immediate problem of social withdrawal, Mary verbalized her fear of an "urinary accident." Following the completion of the first stage of her recent colostomy, she told of the fear that odor might be detected from the colostomy recepticle. She also felt sensitive that the bulge of the colostomy bag could be easily observed. Since completion of the second stage operation, her fears of odors and unsightly bulges remain.

Currently, Mary is seen on a monthly basis or when her feelings of being "bottled up" or of social isolation, or her ambivalence toward her husband, become unbearably strong. She continues to recover muscle tone in her abdomen and has lost five pounds. She is discussing a part-time job, and depending upon her physical stamina, would like to resume part-time work outside the home. Monthly therapeutic contacts are primarily supportive in nature, and the outcome appears closely related to her physical recovery and physical self-image.

The Case of Roberto

Roberto is a 45-year-old comptroller for a large corporation. He is married and is the father of two boys, ages seven and eleven. His wife is a housewife, who sells cosmetics on a part-time basis. He suffers no allergies. Current medication is Zyloprim, which was prescribed after an episode of gout one year ago. Patient also has been taking Milltown for "nerves" for the past two years.

Both of Roberto's parents are living, mother age 72 and father age 74. His father suffers from emphysema and prostate troubles. Economically, Roberto is currently enjoying his greatest success. Five years ago, after serving as an accountant for a firm for over 15 years, he was abruptly terminated. After a period of a year's unemployment, Roberto took a job with his current company, and rose rapidly with the organizational structure. At the age of 17, Roberto was told that he suffered hypothyroidism, but medical tests at the time were not conclusive. History of duodenal ulcer within the past five years. Present problem is the presence of a boil in his external perirectal area.

Physical and Laboratory Workup

Roberto is five feet, eleven and one-half inches and walks with a pronounced slouch. He weighs 172 pounds and has a slight paunch. Blood pressure is 150/110. Sigmoidoscopy revealed a perirectal ulcer. A barium enema was obtained which revealed pilonidal cyst and fistula. Blood studies, urinalysis, and X-rays were within normal limits.

Medical Problem Profile

With Roberto, the following problem listing was developed:

1. Pararectal abscess—Preliminary treatment to consist of drainage under local anesthetic.
2. Hypertension—Revealed in physical workup and sustained in four subsequent observations.
3. Depression and anxiety—Appears to be long-standing.
4. Recurrent episodes of gout.
5. Heavy smoking—Three to four packs of high nicotine cigarettes per day.
6. Excessive alcohol intake—Six plus drinks per day.
7. Dormant duodenal ulcer.
8. Dark mole on back.

Following the drainage of the pararectal abscess, the patient was given instructions concerning diet, urged to switch to lower nicotine cigarettes and to reduce alcohol intake. He indicated a willingness to undertake counseling and was referred to the psychologist.

Personality Profile

On the MMPI, the results shown in Figure 9-2 were obtained.

The elevated F score in this college graduate suggests the high level of stress and the interference that his emotional problems are producing. Clinically, Roberto's profile suggests a modest, sensitive individual with high potential for

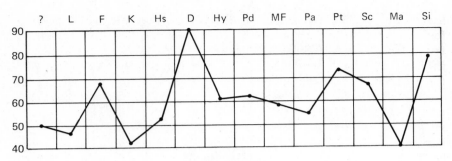

Figure 9–2.

self-dissatisfaction. In addition, Roberto appears as an individual who resists familiarity and maintains a social reserve, is prone to worry, and suffers a variety of depressive and tension symptoms. His problems are likely of long standing, and appear as psychoneurosis, obsessive compulsive type.

Discussion

A total of three interviews were conducted with Roberto. He told of his early childhood, working in a pharmacy owned and operated by his father. He describes his father as one of the most unhappy, most joyless people that he has ever known. His father planned Roberto's life and when Roberto did not select pharmacy as a college major—he chose engineering instead—his father was very upset for years afterward. While away from home attending college, Roberto became interested in aviation and obtained a pilot's license. Roberto encountered difficulty with the engineering curriculum and, upon urging from his advisor, switched to accounting, in which he made very high grades, finally obtaining a B.S. in accounting.

According to Roberto, he has never liked accounting. The attention to details, the need to produce perfect ledgers and reports, creates a deep fear of making an error. He frequently works 12 to 14 hours a day, checking and rechecking his computations before finally submitting a report.

Roberto is married and has two children. He has felt trapped in his profession for the past ten years. When the firm for whom he had worked for 15 years was merged with another firm, he was preemptorily let go, and was unemployed for 12 months, which he described as "the most miserable time in my life."

He then became employed in a company dealing with engineering products, and for the past four years has advanced steadily up the administrative ladder. In analyzing his success on his current job, Roberto attributes much to his immediate supervisor, a vice-president, who is an emotionally warm and open individual with whom the patient has a trusting relationship. During the past year, his firm has expanded its scope of operation with more budgetary and financial decisions forced upon Roberto as comptroller. The feeling of being trapped, the excessive fear of making a mistake, have become stronger, causing him to become more and more compelled to make detailed reports, and to have less and less time for family, social, and recreational activities. Alcohol intake has likewise increased.

Roberto's perfectionist tendencies were discussed in depth during all three interviews. His pararectal abscess again flaired up, and a decision was made for surgical repair. He underwent surgical treatment of what proved to be a fistula-in-ano which ran down into a pilonidal sinus. No complications developed, and he was discharged from the hospital after four days. One week after release from the hospital, Roberto was seen for further discussion of his emotional problems. He reported that the four-day hospitalization gave him an opportunity to think through some of his problems, and in particular his striving, self-dissatisfied nature. He vowed that he was going to make a conscious effort to attempt to ignore minor details and focus on larger accomplishments. While in the hospital, he decided that he and his family should obtain more enjoyment through hobbies and recreational activities. He told the therapist that if things "closed in" on him that he would return.

One year later Roberto made an appointment with the counselor. During the past year he and his family had taken up skiing and tennis. He reported that the vice-president of the firm to whom he felt closeness had died of an apparent heart attack. He felt a deep sense of loss and experienced a recurrence of previous depression and tension.

Three therapeutic sessions were spent in helping Roberto understand and accept the impact of the death of his supervisor-friend. In a telephone followup six months after this last contact, Roberto continues to cope as comptroller in the engineering firm and has been able to delegate some of his duties to other components of the organization.

The Case of Elizabeth

Elizabeth is a 59-year-old housewife married to a truck driver. Her 36-year-old son lives next door, and is engaged in a livestock business. Elizabeth handles much of her son's business at the present time, because her son is in the throes of a divorce. The son's livestock business is marginal, and he drives a school bus part-time for additional funds.

There is diabetes in a maternal cousin. There is no family history of breast cancer, rheumatic fever, heart disease, or TB. Six years ago Elizabeth suffered a duodonal ulcer with no recurrence. A hysterectomy was performed 12 years ago. She does not use alcohol or tobacco, and spends most of her time in household enterprises. The only medication taken is an estrogenic compound and occasional Anacin for arthritis. The reason for seeking medical help is her current mental condition, which Elizabeth describes as "mixed up," "depressed," and "assuming everyone else's problems,"

Physical and Laboratory Workup

Elizabeth stands five feet, four inches, and weighs 152 pounds. Her blood pressure is 138/82, confirmed by three readings. Physical examination revealed an abdominal mass and fibroid tissue in vaginal area, probably result of hysterectomy. Sigmoidscope examination revealed scar tissue in anterior rectal area, no obstructions or inflammations. Several small polyps were also observed. Laboratory findings were negative. Urinalysis reports negative findings for ketones and sugar.

Medical Problem Profile

After obtaining all test results, the physician and Elizabeth developed the following listing of problems:

1. Self dissatisfaction and depression—Inability to enjoy life, chronically worrying over son, her health, her economic situation. Has previously consulted three psychiatrists and two mental health centers.
2. History of stomach ulcer—While not active at this time, this is a concern to patient.
3. Rectal polyps—Minor and should respond to topical applications.
4. Family history of diabetes—Will require annual check.
5. Stress incontinence—Not a major problem, but infrequent occurrences are a source of great concern to the patient.

In the discussion between Elizabeth and the physician, she indicated her willingness to undertake counseling for her emotional problems, and an appointment was made with the psychologist.

Personality Profile

Elizabeth's MMPI profile is shown in Figure 9-3:
Elizabeth's attitude toward answering the questions appears forthright. With the elevations on the clinical scales, it is important to note that her F score is within normal limits, suggesting adequate reality awareness. Her peak elevations on Pd, D, and Pt suggest an individual who has severe internal stress. Problems connected with control of impulses are suggested by the elevated Pd, while exces-

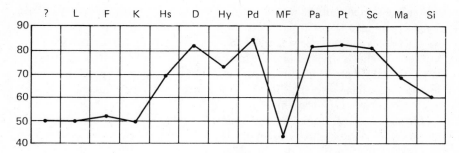

Figure 9–3.

sive concern about the effect of her acts upon others is suggested by elevated D and Pt. Medical patients with such profiles may complain of vague pains, peptic ulcer, headaches. Dependency and insecurity are frequently noted, requiring a great deal of reassurance. In answering specific questions, Elizabeth indicated prior troubles because of sex behavior, vague pains in the head area, possible suicidal thoughts, and fear of losing her mind. In summary, this is a profile of a deeply disturbed person. The differential diagnostic problem is whether this is the profile of a psychotic or a severely neurotic individual. In light of her normal F score, a tentative diagnosis of psychoneurosis, obsessive compulsive type, is warranted.

Discussion

In the initial meeting, Elizabeth appeared relatively calm and her emotional control appeared adequate when obtaining basic case material data. When asked to describe her problems in her own words, she sat back, closed her eyes, and became progressively more and more agitated. She told of her many quests for help over the past ten years. Her last effort was at a mental health center where, after four interviews, she was told that she was a severe obsessive compulsive, and that she must learn to live with her problems. In anticipating this first interview, Elizabeth revealed that she had spent literally hours organizing her life history material.

   She told of her childhood, of being the oldest child with a younger brother. Her father was slow and a perfectionist, and she had a labile, emotional mother who was always physically sick. Elizabeth said that for as long as she can remember, she was actually afraid of her mother, who would become abusive to her at the slightest provocation. Had Elizabeth been growing up today, she would have been labeled an abused child. The mother's behavior toward the brother was protective and overconcerned. After obtaining a high school diploma. Elizabeth took a job in a jewelry store, and was fired for pilfering the cash register. She stated that she was so ashamed and afraid of her mother's reactions that she continued to get dressed each morning and leave the house, so as to give the impression that she was going to work. This continued for two weeks, until the pay check was due, and she had to confess to her parents what had happened at the store. Her mother went into a rage, striking the patient in the mouth and breaking several of her teeth. She was told to leave home and never to return. She was 18 at the time.

Elizabeth vowed, from that date, that she would never make a mistake of any sort again. She obtained employment as a clerk in a department store where she worked for 25 years. At the age of 26, she fell in love with a fellow employee, and while engaged, became pregnant. Her husband-to-be refused to marry her, and she delivered a son and kept him, despite urgings to place him for adoption. At the age of 33, she met her current husband, who accepted both her and her son, and they were married. Her mother has suffered a CVA and is presently in a nursing home.

Her current concerns center around her son and his recent breakup with his common-law wife. His economic problems are "worrying her to death." Elizabeth can recite the actual dates of all of the events of her life—the day, month, and year! She reports severe sleep problems, with nightmares and insomnia. She expresses severe doubt that she can be helped, and the fear that she is only spending her husband's money needlessly. Elizabeth then expressed strong concern that she would become dependent on the therapist. She desires that the therapist give her a list of "dos" and "don'ts" that she must follow. The initial interview confirms the MMPI findings of a severely disturbed woman with many compulsions and obsessions. Her fear of dependency, and her desire for someone to automatically give her a list of rules to follow, typify her dilemma.

Because of her long-standing difficulties and previous inability to gain from psychotherapy, a performance contract was developed. With Elizabeth, it was agreed that she would be seen for four sessions, at which time either the therapist or the patient could terminate future therapy if lack of progress was noted. Using such a technique, if Elizabeth became fearful of dependency upon the therapist or felt that her condition worsened, then contacts would cease. Specific goals to be accomplished during the next four interviews were:

1. The patient would attempt to overcome her fear of germs and only wash her dishes twice instead of the four or five washings that occurred after each meal.
2. The patient would select one activity that previously gave her joy and that she now was not doing, and enter into this activity.
3. She will allow the therapist to stop her rumination of her fears, compulsions, and obsessions during the coming interviews and to switch the subject to other less anxiety-laden subjects.

Elizabeth agreed to this performance contract.

At the end of the four sessions, Elizabeth had succeeded in reducing her dishwashing behavior. The activity she selected was going for a ride in the mountains on Sundays. Two such trips were made, with minimal distress being experienced. As to the content of the interview material, by the fourth session Elizabeth appeared less disturbed when interrupted by the therapist and could shift her attention and focus to other more neutral topics. Before a followup appointment could be made to determine if the therapy should be continued, Elizabeth's mother lapsed into a coma in the nursing home, and subsequently died. Two weeks after the funeral, Elizabeth telephoned the office and said that she was managing her life better, and would not schedule any further appointments at that time. One further contact by Elizabeth occurred with the physician, who prescribed medication to help her sleep.

Certainly her prognosis is not good. Her adjustment for the past 15 years has been marginal at best. Whether she will return or not remains to be seen. Her history of "doctor shopping" suggests that she most likely has sought medical help elsewhere in the six months that have passed since her last contact.

Summary

Psychoneuroses, when encountered in a general medical setting, are in many ways similar to chronic diseases such as arthritis. Within the patients's total medical constellation of physical, emotional, evnironmental, and social concerns, the pain generated by neuroses will fluctuate considerably. In the three cases presented, the neurotic components have been present for many years, and have been resistant to prior therapeutic efforts. Brief psychotherapy/counseling could not be expected to eradicate such pains, but can be utilized as an educational effort to enable the patient to cognitively better understand the physiological and emotional side effects of his disease. With Mary, Roberto, and Elizabeth, deep and intensive psychotherapy would propbably be required before substantial change could be noted in their behavior and emotions. The cost of such treatment and the commitment by the patient to such long term efforts are realistic factors in referring psychoneurotic patients for deeper, more intensive care. All three of the patients included as case material were aware that many of their difficulties could be attributed to emotional problems. One, Elizabeth, had actively sought help from a variety of sources. Lack of available treatment resources, fear of openly seeking mental health care, or lack of financial resources to undertake such treatment caused each patient to bring his problems to his family practitioner. Through the combined approach of the problem-oriented medical record coupled with minimal psychodiagnostic procedures, a fuller picture of the patient's emotional-physical interactions can be obtained. Through the combined knowledge of the physician and psychologist, brief psychotherapy and crisis support can be offered by both physician and psychologist.

References

1. Masserman, Jules H. *The Practice of Dynamic Psychiatry*. Philadelphia: W.B. Saunders Co., 1955, p. 124.

2. Freud, S. *Collected Papers, Vol. II*. London: Hogarth Press, 1924, p. 256.

10 Borderline Psychotic States in General Medical Practice

An individual's mental activity is expressed in four main aspects—what he *does* (behaviorally), what he *says* (verbally), how he *feels* (inferred from speech and actions), and what and how he *thinks* (conveyed primarily through speech). In the chapter dealing with psychoneuroses, by definition these are "functional" disorders of *feelings* that indirectly affect actions and thoughts. In psychotic or psychoticlike states, the changes in thought and feeling become so intense that all spheres of mental activity become altered—thinking, reasoning, behavior, as well as feelings. In a psychotic state, the patient's sense of values may be seriously altered, his perceptions of the world may differ radically from those around him, he may or may not be aware that something strange is occurring within him, and he may speak a different language from those around him.

Too often in the literature, it is implied that an individual suffering emotional problems is either suffering a psychosis or a psychoneurosis. One frequently sees an individual under observation slip from a psychoneurotic state into a psychotic state or vice versa, just as has been observed with "normals" who under stress begin to exhibit psychoneurotic symptoms. The clear demarcation lines between a severe psychoneurosis and a psychoticlike state often depend upon the particular time at which the patient is observed. One of the clinical cases included is that of Steve, who at first examination appeared to be suffering a psychoneurotic type of adjustment, and a year leater, exhibited full psychological, behavioral, and thinking disorders comparable to a psychotic state.

Thoughts, in a psychotic state, may take on the characteristics of an hallucination. The patient, in attempting to find a logical and/or rational reason for his or her strange behavior, may concoct an elaborate and complicated "explanation" to account for such feelings or behavior. In some psychotic states, memory or time distortions may occur. Four major groupings of psychoses are generally accepted:[1]

1. **Affective disorders.** Individuals who exhibit striking increases in feeling tones such as elation, anger, fear, depression, or anxiety are suffering from the manic-depressive psychosis. Such affective states are of such an extreme on either the

elation end of the continuum or the depression end of the continuum that behavior, thinking, and/or reasoning are impaired. Usually such attacks are cyclical in nature, usually of a self-limited nature. Research suggest that age of onset is significantly related to affective psychoses.[2] Rarely is a true case of affective psychosis found below the age of 35 years. Manic-depressive psychosis is primarily a middle-aged phenomenon. Constitutional factors have been shown to play a part in the affective disorders.[3] A detailed history of prior mood swings, the context of feelings and thoughts are the areas of intensive investigation in attempting to assess the presence or absence of an affective psychoses.

2. Schizophrenic disorders. The derivation of the word "schizo" suggests the splitting off or fragmentation of aspects of the thinking or emotions of the sufferer. "Phrenic," on the other hand, suggests a return to a childlike state. Current clinical thinking tends to the view that there are many kinds of schizophrenias.

Paranoid disorders are likely of long duration and are characterized by an intellectual system of delusions and possibly hallucinations. An individual picked up by police for shooting out electrical transformers who explains that the FBI is beaming radio impulses and attempting to influence his thoughts is an example of an intellectualized delusional system. The higher the intellectual ability of the sufferer of paranoid schizophrenia, the more rational and logical such delusional systems appear. Intellectual deterioration, if present, is usually a slow process.

Simple schizophrenia is usually evidenced by a blunting of emotional feelings, lack of initiative, apathy, and inability to plan for the future. Thinking distortions are evident, but sufferers do not demonstrate delusional or hallucinatory thinking. A detailed history of an individual suffering this form of schizophrenia usually shows a slow and insidious process with no observable stress points from which radical changes of behavior can be attributed.

Hebephrenic schizophrenia is characterized by childishness in behavior, speech, and emotions; silliness; and regressions to earlier stages of adjustment, as well as bizarre delusions and hallucinations. Irreversible intellectual deterioration may be rapid.

Catatonic schizophrenia is characterized by the patient's mobility and activity level. Stuporous, mute, inactive, taking no interest in immediate surroundings, or refusal to eat, interrupted by periods of excitement, are symptoms of this form of schizophrenia.

As with the affective psychoses, schizophrenic reactions appear to have a genetic or constitutional component.[4]

3. Paranoid disorders. A small percentage of the psychiatric population evidences delusions and hallucinations that are less grotesque than those of paranoid schizophrenics, and show little or no intellectual deterioration over time. The mood of such a patient is usually in keeping with the content of his delusion. Suspiciousness and hatred may be evident if the delusional state is one of persecution. Expansiveness and grandiosity may be present if the delusional system centers around the exalted state of the sufferer—i.e., the belief that he is the heir of a vast fortune. Due to the rarity of this condition, and the difficulty in differentiating this disorder from a schizophrenic process, final diagnosis will usually not occur in an outpatient setting. When encountering individual patients with paranoidlike features, the physician will be forced to interpret and explain all procedures, and document through records that such interpretations have been made. In one pending malpractice suit with which the author is acquainted, the man contemplating the malpractice suit is being urged on by his wife, who appears to demonstrate many paranoidlike features.

4. Organic psychoses. As a result of structural disease or injury to the brain by trauma or toxaemia, individuals may evidence impairment or clouding of the intellect or emotions. Orientation to time and place, memory gaps, impaired reasoning and comprehension, and changing ethical and moral standards suggest the degrees of impairment. Along with such impairment, there may be efforts by the patient to "confabulate" the memory gaps by attempting to make up a plausible explanation. Delusions, false perceptions, or hallucinations may also be present. Some organic psychoses may be acute states such as toxic-exhaustive states, while others such as arteriosclerotic dementia may be chronic. Incidence of organic psychoses are usually age-related, occurring in middle and later life. In recent years, with increased ingestion of drugs among the young, the potential diagnosis of organic psychoses cannot be reserved for only the aged.

Due to the physiological and organic aspects of this category of psychoses, inpatient diagnoses and treatment are mandatory.

In a general outpatient medical setting, occurrences of psychotic episodes are rarely seen. In inpatient settings, following surgery, anesthesia, or severe accidents, elements of temporary psychotic reactions can be observed. Usually such reactions are short-lived and related to physical recovery, and the patient returns to the prehospitalization adjustment level. Drug ingestion in the youth culture also presents symptoms similar to schizophrenia.

Because of the potential danger of the psychosis, primarily to the patient, outpatient treatment is rarely the treatment of choice in a general medical setting. Two of the illustrative cases contained in this chapter were obtained from inpatient consultations. The third case is illustrative of a class of younger patients who present a curious mixture of psychoneurotic-psychotic-character disorders. Unfortunately, with the institutional and social revolutions that are occurring among younger generations, it seems likely that such "mixed" types of maladjustments will be on the increase and that the general practitioner will find more of his younger patients exhibiting such behavioral and emotional characteristics.

The Case of Susan

This 32-year-old housewife was accompanied to the physician's office by her husband. She refused to go into the examining room alone, and insisted that her husband go with her. When the physician attempted to ask her reason for seeking medical attention, she turned to her husband and said, "Ask him, it's his idea." Susan's husband related that they had just moved to the area from Kansas several months ago with their three children, ages two, four, and six years. Since the move, he reports that Susan is "just not feeling well." She sleeps 10 to 14 hours per day, and remains in bed complaining of tiredness and exhaustion. She is not maintaining her home, and her attention to the children's needs is minimal. Prior medical history includes appendectomy at age 18. The patient was told that she suffered from anemia while in Kansas. One year prior to leaving Kansas, Susan had suffered a "nervous breakdown," and was hospitalized in the state hospital for several months. The husband attributes her "breakdown" to a family argument between Susan and her parents, upon whom she had been extremely dependent all of her life. During her husband's description of her past history, Susan sat passively in the chair, motionless, not once entering into the conversation or supplying information. Susan showed no signs of happiness, sadness, or alertness, and appeared oblivious to her surroundings. At this point, the physician recommended that Susan be hospitalized in the local general hospital. The husband turned to Susan and said "What about that, Hon?" to which Susan merely shrugged her shoulders and said nothing.

Physical and Laboratory Workup

Upon admission to the hospital, the patient's height was recorded as five feet, two and one-half inches; weight, 112 pounds. Blood pressure was 110/73. When an attempt was made to draw blood for laboratory study, Susan reacted violently, refusing to cooperate in any way, accusing the technician and the ward nurses of attempting to dope her and control her mind. At this point the physician was notified of her combative attitude. A consultation was requested by the psychologist.

Personality Profile

On her first day in the hospital, Susan was seen by the psychologist, who asked her to complete the MMPI. In response to this request, Susan made no indication as to whether she would comply. The MMPI questionnaire and pencil were placed in front of her on a bed table and the psychologist left the room. Nursing personnel were asked to encourage Susan to complete the questionnaire. Four hours later Susan completed the MMPI.

The results of the MMPI are shown in Figure 10-1.

The exceedingly elevated F score indicates poor contact with reality. Peak scores on schizophrenia and depression at T scores exceeding 90 is rare in normal subjects. Responses to individual items suggest that Susan is fearful of losing her mind, hears voices when alone, has a feeling that things are not real, and apparently suspects that someone is attempting to influence her mind. In addition, Susan indicates that most of the time she wishes she was dead. Susan appears to be suffering a form of schizophrenia with hallucinations and delusions.

Discussion

In further discussion with her husband, he supplied additional information. Susan and her husband have been married seven years. When her husband first met Susan, at 22, she was exceedingly shy, having very few contacts. The husband met her through an older brother. While in high school, she developed a fear of crowds, dropping out of high school in her junior year despite an almost straight A academic record. Following her marriage, she delivered three children without incident, and seemingly built her life around the care of the children. Her current ignoring of the children is the most puzzling aspect of Susan's sickness to her husband.

Approximately 14 months ago, while her husband was at work, Susan barricaded herself in her bedroom, refusing to allow anyone to enter. She could be heard talking and screaming obscenities. The local physician was called, the door removed from its hinges, and a massive tranquilizer administered. The physician recommended that Susan be admitted to the state mental hospital,

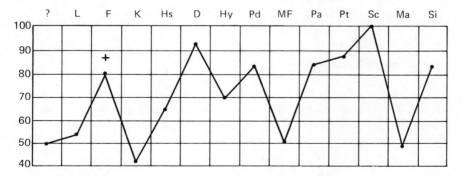

Figure 10-1.

which was done. For the first three months Susan refused to see her husband or immediate family. The husband does not know the form of treatment Susan received, but believes only drug therapy was used. After approximately six months, Susan appeared to be recovering, and began to beg her husband to bring her home. Against medical advice and "because the children needed her so much," her husband succumbed to her wishes. Adjustment at home, according to the husband, was about the way it had always been until three weeks ago. At that time she withdrew, appeared to want to sleep all day and stay up all night. She became secretive and bizarre in her behavior.

In direct interview with Susan, she admitted that someone was attempting to control her mind and thoughts. She thought it was some sort of a radar or electrical transmission. After discussing her fears and conclusions, she suddenly asked "How do I know you aren't one of them?" and refused to talk. Arrangements were made for Susan to be transferred to a private psychiatric facility.

The Case of Steven

This 39-year-old furniture salesman was referred to the physician-surgeon by the emergency room of the general hospital, because of rectal bleeding. Steven has been married to his third wife for nine years, and there are no children. Steven is a Korean War veteran. Born and reared in Chicago, the third child of a large Roman Catholic family, he migrated to the area six years ago. He describes himself as always being a nervous, high strung person, who has difficulty understanding why individuals do not have more concern for others. Both of Steven's parents are living and apparently in good health. There is no family history of cancer, heart disease, rheumatic fever, or diabetes. Two of Steven's siblings have been diagnosed as suffering hypoglycemia. For several years, Steven has suffered intermittent pains in bowel elimination with soilage. Exterior hemorrhoids have occurred and were treated by the patient with patent medicine remedies. A previous operation for hemorrhoid disease had been performed three years ago.

Physical and Laboratory Workup

Steven stands six feet, one inch, and weighs 202 pounds. Blood pressure is 120/70. Physical examination revealed no gross abnormalities. Patient is slightly obese. His testicles appear smaller than normal. Blood studies reveal no abnormalities. Sigmoidoscopy reveals hemorrhoid disease with condyloma accuminata and a suspected fistula-in-ano. Because of the discomfort and the desire of the patient to have his rectal problems corrected, an operation was scheduled for the following week. A tentative medical problem profile was developed.

Medical Problem Profile

Problem No. 1. Recurrent hemorrhoid disease—surgery required
Problem No. 2. Anxiety and hyperactivity
Problem No. 3. Heavy smoking—over two packs per day for years
Problem No. 4. Mild obesity

Steven was admitted to the general hospital with a preoperative diagnosis of hemorrhoid disease with condyloma accuminatum. The surgery was performed without incident. The surgical findings and procedures were:

Findings: There was a heavy and luxuriant growth of condylomata for about 3 or 4 cms around the anus. It did not appear that there were any condylomata above the dentate line. The anal lining was very thick and scarred. The patient had had a previous hemorrhoidectomy but the type could not be determined. There were huge amonts of varicosities most prominent in the right and left lateral and dorsal aspects and a moderate amount anteriorly. This tissue was very much involved with scar and large veins. In addition, there was a T-shaped fistula-in-ano coming up dorsally in the muscle and the limbs of the T growing left and right. It was this aspect which undoubtedly accounted for his soilage and bleeding as the sphincter really could not function.

Surgical Procedures: Sigmoidoscopy was performed the length of the scope. The rectal mucosa was normal. Dorsal sphincterotomy was performed. Slivers of mucosa were removed laterally. Extensive and bloody dissection resulted in a loss of 350 ccs of blood during the operation and the removal of large amounts of submucosal scar in the whole circumference of the anus and the release of the contractures dorsally. Some of the anal lining was also removed. Bleeding was controlled chiefly with electrocautery and some fine plain catgut. At the end of the surgery the electrocautery was used to systematically fulgurate the condylomata and these were then shaved off. Care was taken not to destroy too much perianal skin. A Xylocaine visous apparatus, pressure dressing was applied and the patient returned to the recovery room in good condition.

Five days later, the patient was discharged, bowels moving normally and eating was normal. Outpatient treatment was continued for treatment of condylomata and postoperative care.

In his first postoperative outpatient visit, Steven discussed his nervousness with the physician and asked for help. A referral was made for Steven to be seen by the psychologist. Prior to this appointment, Steven completed the MMPI.

Personality Profile

The elevated F score shown in Figure 10-2 suggests the seriousness of Steven's emotional conflict. Individuals with peaks on depression and psychopathic

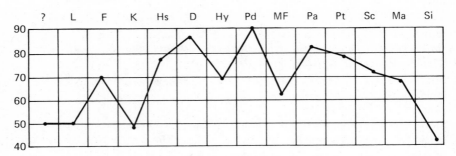

Figure 10–2.

deviate scales tend to have long-standing behavioral problems: alcoholism and disrupted relations with the opposite sex are common. Irritability, suspiciousness, and depression may also be present.

In response to critical items, this patient indicates fear of losing his mind, a feeling that his sins are unpardonable, admits excessive use of alcohol, and a feeling of constant anxiety. Elements of psychoticlike behavior are suggested from the MMPI profile, occurring with suicidal thoughts.

Discussion

Steven was seen for four interviews, and a more detailed social history was obtained. Through his mother's influence, the church was a significant factor in his early life. He served as an altar boy for years. His father was a heavy drinker, which led to much interfamily turmoil during Steven's childhood. When Steven was 17, his father deserted his mother and went to live with another woman. Steven and his siblings were very divided in their attitudes toward the father, most of them overtly hating the father. Steven described his reaction as attempting to maintain a "Christian view" toward his father. At age 18 he entered the army, more to get away from the family arguments than for any other reason. In the army he became depressed, drank excessively, and made a suicide attempt. Upon discharge from the Army, he was confined in a Veteran's Administration psychiatric facility for eight months. In describing his sickness, he said it was "like he built a wall around himself." He heard voices, mostly relating spiritual messages. He said at the depth of his illness, people would attempt to talk to him and he could not hear them, only see their lips move. His discharge from the VA hospital occurred with the help of his father, who got him a job in a furniture store and encouraged his "getting back into the world." While working as a furniture salesman, he was married twice, both marriages ending in divorce and producing no children. Neither marriage was performed in the church.

Six months ago his father's common-law wife died. The father promptly returned to Steven's mother, and was completely accepted by her. Steven suffers from tremendous ambivalence toward his father. The father visited Steven and his third wife (this marriage was performed in a church) a month prior to surgery. The father continues to drink heavily and succeeded in getting himself and the patient intoxicated. Steven came to his senses on a bus, accompanying his father, who had talked Steven into going to California with him. Steven left his father and returned home, very guilt-laden and hating himself for being "taken in" by his father. Three sessions were spent is discussing his feelings of ambivalence toward his father. Steven talked at length of his conflict between religious attitudes and his personal attitudes toward his father and mother. Steven's depression abated and he said he felt that he could handle these feelings by himself. A good relationship was established with Steven and he was encouraged to return if he felt he needed help.

Ten months later, on a Sunday morning, Steven's wife called the therapist to say that Steven had been drinking heavily and was talking of committing suicide. She wanted Steven hospitalized for his own safety. She said that Steven had asked her to call the therapist, and to have him arrange hospitalization. The local VA hospital was contacted and a bed was reportedly available. Steven accompanied by his wife, waited eight hours at the VA hospital, and then was told that no bed was available. He was referred to the emergency room of the local general hospital. At the emergency room, the psychologist and physician were again contacted, and arrangements were made for Steven to be placed in a single room until further arrangements for inpatient psychiatric hospitalization could be made. Thorozine 150 mg. per day was immediately administered.

Inpatient Personality Profile

Eight hours after this emergecy hospitalization, a second MMPI was obtained, represented in Figure 10–3 by the solid line. The profile obtained ten months before is indicated by the dotted line.

Contrasting Steven's present profile with the results obtained ten months previously, slippage in reality awareness has occurred (F). Depression is higher now than previously, but Pd–acting out behavior appears to have diminished. The outstanding changes in the ten month interval are the tremendous increases in Sc and Pt scales. From these results, it would appear that Steven has suffered a schizophrenic break, and the profiles actually demonstrate the eruption of a schizophrenic psychosis. The presence or absence of hallucinations and/or delusions will be keys to assessing the degree of this psychotic eruption.

Meanwhile, difficulties were encountered in obtaining a psychiatric placement for Steven and it was decided to institute a series of inpatient tests. Steven's desire was to remain in the general hospital, and not go into a psychiatric facility. Neurologic and internal medicine consultation was requested.

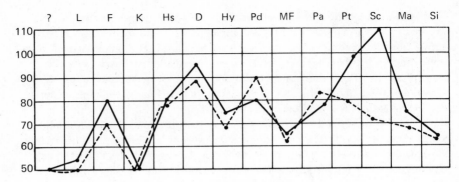

Figure 10–3.

Neurologic Findings (Four days after emergency hospitalization): The patient is a tall, slightly overweight young man who is alert and oriented. He appears to have a somewhat offhand joking manner. His gait is not wide-based or disequilibrated and he walks tandum reasonably well. There was no sysphagia or dysarthria and the neck seems supple. The pupils are round, regular, and equal, and react to light and accommodation. The visual fields are full to confrontation. The patient may have early papilledema in that the optic disc margins were slightly indistinct and the veins appear to be somewhat fuller than normal, although there does appear to be a reasonably well-preserved optic cup. There is a slight ptosis of the left upper eyelid. There is no impairment to light touch, pin prick over the face and there is no facial weakness. Hearing is intact to the tuning fork. There was no nystagmus. The palate is symmetrical. There appears to be a mild elective weakness on the left, somewhat more evident in the leg than arm. There is some impairment to rapidly alternating movements with both hands and a moderate intension tremor and ataxia with the left arm. (The patient is on Thorazine and this may not be a valid finding at the present time.) The deep tendon reflexes are quite sluggish but symmetrical. The plantar response is sluggish bilaterally. The superficial abdominal reflexes are present at a trace in all four quadrants. The skull X-ray were seen and revealed slight shift of the pinea from right to left. Echoencephalogram has been performed, but results are not yet available.

Impression: 1) Depressive reaction, severe
2) Rule out brain tumor, right frontal lobe

Recommendations: I believe this patient should also have a brain scan and if this suggests any abnormalities, an angiography or CAT scan.

Internal Medicine Findings: A lower than normal serum testosterone is present. Thyroid function is entirely normal. During hospitalization he was observed to drink huge quantities of water. Urinalysis reveals entirely normal findings. EKG and chest X-ray are normal. Slight deviation in pinea already noted. Upper barium X-rays suggest small hiatus hernia. Brain scan revealed no abnormalities. Appears to be acute depressive reaction, cause undetermined.

Psychological Findings

Steven remained secluded with his door closed most of the time during his first four days in the hospital. He related that this was because he didn't want anyone to see him cry. Without provocation, he would suddenly become tearful, chastising himself for being "weak" and "stupid" when this occurred.

In filling in events during the past ten months since he was last seen, Steven revealed that, against his better judgment, he went back to Chicago for the Christmas holidays. The old hatreds, ambivalences, and despair centering around his love-hate attitudes toward his father emerged during his stay. Overindulgence in alcohol was his method of coping. His wife confirmed his reactions; after seven days in Chicago, Steven was a "nervous wreck" according to his wife.

Upon his return home after the family visit, Steven's mood kept sinking lower and lower. Alcohol no longer enabled him to put these thoughts out of his mind. Insomnia increased. At the time he called asking for inpatient treatment he was at the "end of his rope."

Four sessions were spent with Steven, encouraging him to express his feelings rather than what he *thought* he should feel. On the sixth day in the hospital, he began to open his door and to talk and kid with the nurses. He reported to the psychologist that he had "turned the corner." When asked to explain, he said that after thinking about all his guilts, and his lack of understanding of his father and mother, he had decided that he was spinning his wheels pondering such things, because he could do nothing about their lives.

From that point, he became more outgoing. Fits of despondency ceased. His wife noted his change in behavior. Plans to have him enter an inpatient psychiatric facility were canceled.

In a staff conference nine days after emergency hospitalization, he was released from the hospital, and continues to take 150 mgs. of Thorazine per day. He returned to work a week after release and continues to receive biweekly outpatient care by both physician and psychologist.

The Case of Nell

Nell is a 21-year-old single girl who has dropped out of college after three rather unaffecting years which she did not enjoy. There are two older brothers, ages 27 and 25. Her hobby is walking by herself in the mountains, enjoying nature. She is not employed. Nell, a daughter of a present patient, sought medical attention because of intermittent bilateral chest pains. Medication history includes Ovulen-21 for the past three years, Valium, Thorazine for three months while at college, APC with codein. Previous surgeries include tonsillectomy and adenoidectomy at age five. Patient was in automobile accident in

1972, injuring a knee. There is a family history of diabetes in both maternal and paternal grandparents.

Physical and Laboratory Findings

Nell is five feet, seven inches tall and weighs 125 pounds. Blood pressure is 120/60. Physical examination of G.I., G.U., lymphatics, neuromuscular, and skin reveal no abnormalities. Blood studies and urinalysis reveal no abnormalities—EKG, chest X-rays, negative. Serum calcium found negative. Estrogen found negative. Estrogen normal. Upon completion of the medical workup, Nell and the physician developed the following medical problem profile.

Medical Problem Profile

Problem No. 1. Chest pain—present for last three months
Problem No. 2. Premenstrual swelling—weight gain of three to four pounds, breast enlargement, irritability
Problem No. 3. Social dissociation—reports "nervous breakdown" five months prior; crying, depressed, poor response to psychiatric treatment
Problem No. 4. Chrondo-malacia patellae, bi-lateral—has full range of motion but stands with curved legs

During the physical and consultation with Nell, it was observed that her tension level and mood varied greatly when she was seen alone or with her mother. When asked, in the presence of her mother, if she desired counseling for some of her emotional and "nervous" problems, Nell acted very nonchalant, replying "Shrinks don't help—they never did before." Alone with the physician, however, Nell expressed a desire to seek help.

Personality Profile

With the F score shown in Figure 10–4 completely off a scale, an indication was obtained of the severity of Nell's problems. Adjectives such as "odd," "peculiar," "queer," "unpredictable," "impulsive," "nonconforming," and "nomadic," are used to describe individuals with similar profiles. Presence of depression in such a schizoidlike person is of concern because of suicidal possibilities. Individual responses to MMPI items suggest that Nell is dissatisfied with her sexual life, has had past difficulties because of sexual behavior, and has indulged in unusual sex activities. She indicates a wanderlust, a feeling that she is being

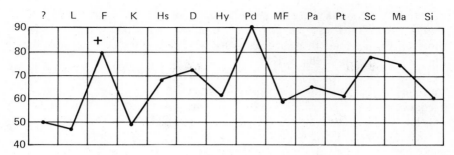

Figure 10-4.

plotted against, and admits that she has strange and peculiar thoughts. She indicated that she sometimes feels as if she must injure herself or others.

The bizarre mixture of lack of impulse control, depression, and schizoid-like responses coupled with the extreme elevated F suggest that Nell is bordering on being out of contact with reality.

Discussion

In the initial interview, Nell came into the room like a wary animal. She began the conversation by saying that she has an animallike sense that could tell her if people "gave her bad vibes." When asked if the psychologist "gave her bad vibes," she said she didn't think so. She was dressed in old, tattered blue jeans with a man's shirt, heavy work boots, and a heavy shapeless mackinaw jacket. When asked how she might be helped, she launched into a monologue, describing how she would like to live like the mountain men of the eighteenth century. She related that she was happiest when totally alone, with no people to "hassle" her. She discussed the ills that man had inflicted upon the environment, and the innate wisdom of animals. Her best friend, according to Nell, is her dog, and is the only creature with whom she can communicate.

She is currently living at home with her mother and father, after dropping out of college four months ago. She rationalizes that she is living at home in order "to help with the housework while her mother has an operation." (It is true that her mother is scheduled for corrective surgery, but concern for Nell on the part of her parents appears the chief reason for her residing at home.)

In attempting to obtain a social history, Nell reported that her adjustment difficulties began in junior high school. She was a runaway, was kept in the detention center on several occasions, experimented with all forms of hard and soft drugs, and currently smokes "pot" once or twice a week. Throughout her life, according to Nell, her troubles and conflicts have vacillated between trying

to please people, particularly her parents, and doing "what is the real me."
Acting out her impulses brings self-satisfaction, but such acts create hurt among
those who love her and then she feels guilty. This pattern has been her style of
life for ten years, according to Nell.

While a junior in high school, and labeled as a delinquent, a woman physical education teacher took a personal interest in Nell and encouraged her to
become a swimmer. She became quite proficient and trained rigorously, stop-
ping her smoking, drinking, pot smoking, and promiscuous sexual behavior. Her
parents were pleased with her change in behavior. Her academic grades improved,
and she became an honor student in her senior year. With encouragement from
her parents, which Nell now interprets as pressure, she agreed to enroll in
college.

Nell changed her major five times in her three years in college. She states
that in the last two years she did nothing but "party." She relates that in the
last year "bed hopping" had been her chief enjoyment. On only one occasion
has she achieved orgasm. During the last year, she says she has been engaged to
be married four times. When asked if she had ever truly loved someone, she
replied that she did love one boy, but they could not get along because both
were so moody and withdrawn. At the conclusion of the first interview, she
stated that her "vibes" were good, and that she thought that the psychologist
was really interested in her. A second appointment was scheduled and Nell
was told that it would be the psychologist's turn to discuss with her the results
of her MMPI.

She arrived 20 minutes late for the second interview. The impulse control
problems suggested in her MMPI were interpreted, along with the depressive
trends. She began to cry when asked what she feels depressed about. While
crying, she stated that she hates to cry, because it makes her feel so weak.
When told that many women cry, she immediately became angry, and said
that she hated being a woman. She then told how, all her life, she felt pressured
by her parents to be a "frilly, silly little girl," when her pleasure and joys came
from playing and entering into activities with her older brothers.

When it was discussed that her conflict between "being herself" and attempting to conform to the expectations of others who love her appeared to
be a problem (almost her exact words from the first interview), she became
sullen, and asked, "You aren't going to try to change my basic values, are you?"
When told that the psychologist didn't know what her basic values were as yet,
she one more launched into her worship of nature, her belief that animal instinct
was more meaningful than man's intellect.

It was suggested that if her position of "wanting to be herself," if it included
acting out all her impulses and desires, was *really* her code of ethics, then some
compromise would have to occur if she was to avoid the guilt and pain that such
actions would cause. She responded to this by saying she would never abandon
her own attitudes of what was "right." The interview closed on this theme, with

Nell being asked to think things over, and at least to consider the possiblity that she might be happier by reconsidering some of her absolute standards. No further contacts have been scheduled by Nell.

The untenable position that Nell has worked herself into, rigidly striving to be true to her own impulses no matter whom she hurts and at the same time feeling guilt over the pain that she causes people who care about her, is a crisis that Nell does not seem to be able to resolve. Whether nomadism—living as a "mountain man"—will win out, or whether Nell will turn potential self-destructive forces upon herself, remains to be seen. In either event, the prognosis is not good.

Summary

When a full-blown psychotic reaction is encountered in a general medical patient, in almost every instance this should be considered a psychiatric emergency. Hodges has listed five conditions to guide the physician in determining if indeed a psychiatric emergency does exist:[5]

1. The patient is disturbed to the extent that he is judged to represent a danger to himself or others.
2. The condition must have arisen suddenly or unexpectedly.
3. Circumstances require immediate action to prevent serious consequences (the patient must be protected from himself or others must be protected from him).
4. A mode of action or treatment is known and available and this treatment must be able to minimize or prevent the potential harmful effects.
5. There must be no contraindication to treatment on an emergency basis.

The three cases presented provide a range of psychotic or psychoticlike reactions found in medical practice. Susan, from the history obtained from her husband, had probably never fully recovered from a severe psychotic episode a year ago. The potential danger that Susan represents to herself and her children mitigated that emergency intervention be undertaken. Accordingly, the general hospital was utilized as the first stage in ultimately getting Susan into a psychiatric facility.

Steven's case represents s typical crisis situation in which the primary physician often finds himself involved. With a long history of psychiatric illness, Steven's sudden change from marginal adjustment to threatening suicide demanded that inpatient treatment be obtained. Unfortunately, arrangements for emergency inpatient psychiatric hospitalization take time. In the interim, some safe environment is required to protect the patient from himself. Again, the utilization of the general medical hospital was the only alternative available.

Steven's speedy remission in the general hospital, and his immediate response to treatment, indicated that the more protective environment of an inpatient psychiatric facility was not demanded.

Nell's case is perhaps the most difficult to deal with on a general medical basis. Prior attempts to convince Nell and her parents that more intensive psychiatric help was needed have been rejected. No overt psychotic behavior was evident, but there were many symptoms of illogical thinking, impulsiveness and paranoidlike attitudes. One has the feeling of sitting on a psychiatric time bomb that could explode at the slightest provocation. Yet, in this instance, both the primary care physician and the psychologist have done their best. Until Nell accepts the responsibility of her own state of health, or until her behavior becomes so deviant as to come into conflict with the law, little can be done. In the meantime, the primary care physician continues to treat Nell for her chest pains, premenstrual weight gains, and other physical emergencies.

References

1. Skottowe, Ian. *Clinical Psychiatry for Practitioners and Students*. New York: McGraw-Hill, 1954, pp. 22–25.

2. Mendels, M.D., and Hawkins, D.R. Sleep Studies in Depression. In *Recent Advances in the Psychobiology of the Depressive Illnesses*. Process, sponsored by The Clinical Research Branch, Division of Extramural Research Programs, National Institute of Mental Health, DHEW Publication No. 70, 9053, 1972, pp. 147–70.

3. Kallmann, F. Genetic Aspects of Psychoses. In *Biology of Mental Health and Disease*. New York: Milbank Memorial Fund, 1952, pp. 283–302.

4. Ibid.

5. Hodges, James R. *Practical Psychiatry for the Primary Physician*. Chicago: Nelson-Hall Publishers, 1975, pp. 309–10.

11 The Domain of Health

In the preceding chapters an effort has been made to integrate the physical/
biolgoical with the emotional/behavioral aspects of health. Hopefully, a con-
vincing rationale has been developed to support the view that a realistic concept
of health must include both facets. The primary care physician, as he or she
assumes the role of the general medical patient's health advocate and advisor,
will, of necessity, be drawn into the emotional/behavioral life areas of the patient. Kass amplifies upon this future role and the implications for the practice
of medicine.

Though health is a natural norm, and though nature provides us with powerful
inborn means of preserving and maintaining a well-working wholeness, it is
wrong to assume that health is the result largely of accident or of external in-
vasion. In the case of non-human animals, such a view could perhaps be de-
fended. Other animals instinctively eat the right foods (when available) and
act in such a way as to maintain their naturally given state of health and vigor.
Other animals do not overeat, undersleep, knowingly ingest toxic substances or
permit their bodies to fall into disuse through sloth, watching T.V. and riding in
automobiles, transacting business, or writing articles about health. For us
human beings, however, even a healthy nature must be nurtured, and maintained
by effort and discipline if it is not to become soft and weak and prone to illness,
and certain excesses and stresses must be avoided if this softness is not to spawn
overt unhealth and disease. One should not, of course, underestimate the role of
germs and other hostile agents working from without; but I strongly suspect
that the germ theory of disease has been oversold, and that the state of "host"
resistance," and in particular of the immunity systems, will become increasingly
prominent in our understanding of both health and disease.
  One the distinction is made between health nurture and maintenance, on the
one hand, and disease prevention and treatment, on the other, it becomes immediately clear that bodily health does not depend only on the body and its
parts. It depends decisively on the psyche with which the body associates and
cooperates. . . . In a most far-reaching way, our health is influenced by our temperament, our character, our habits, our whole way of life. This fact was once
better appreciated than it is today.[1]

Using Kass' distinction between health nurture and disease treatment/
prevention, the primary physician must increase his competency in health-

111

nurturing and health maintenance activities. When encountering a patient suffering the pain of a depression, marital problems, grief, or loneliness, both health-nurturing and disease treatment/prevention approaches often are required. In order to begin even a rudimentary sorting out of the very complex interactions of health nurture–disease prevention needs of the general medical patient, a systematic approach such as POMIS is essential.

It is a basic hypothesis of this book that within every individual at any stage in his life there exists a range of health problems or potential health problems. Some of these problems may be disease-related and require direct treatment intervention. Other health needs may lie in the health nurture realm and dictate that the patient be encouraged to assume personal responsibility for enhancing his own state of health through sensible dietary and alcohol intake, refraining from smoking, and counteracting boredom and depression. If such health nurturance is ignored, full-blown medical conditions can and do develop. The cooperation, understanding, and commitment of the patient to assume responsibility for his health state is crucial if health nurturing is to have a successfull outcome. To better understand the personality makeup of the patient, his temperament, values, and style of life, utilization of personality measures such as the MMPI take on added meaning and are important steps in the primary physician's health-nurturing efforts.

Integrating psychodiagnostic information into the patient's medical history, physical, and laboratory findings provides the necessary data base to better treat overt health problems, as well as clues as to how health nurturance might best be accomplished. Brief counseling or psychotherapy/psychosocial counseling is a natural outgrowth of such an approach.

What happens if the primary physician chooses, either consciously or unconsciously, to ignore the patient's feelings, emotions, temperament, or personal problems, and elects only to deal with complaints of a physical nature? There is some evidence to substantiate the view that patients quickly learn to somatize their personal problems, relating only the physical concomitants to their emotional/behavioral problems, which are then rewarded and reinforced by the attention and concern of the disease-oriented physician.[2] If health nurturance, particularly in the emotional/behavioral areas, is ignored by primary physicians, there are a host of other less qualified sources to which the patient can turn.

If one accepts that many of today's major health problems lie within the temperaments, habits, values, and styles of life of individuals, then it follows that the patient, more than the physician, actually controls his health destiny. One of the major challenges of the primary physician in the future will be how to help patients assume the responsibility for their inner feelings of health and well-being, as well as for their overt behaviors as represented by their habits of work, lovemaking, and recreation. Research suggests that general medical patients are notoriously lax in following medical advice. Approximately 44 percent of general medical patients tend to ignore the health prescriptions and advice given by thier physicians.[3] Many factors may be contributing to such findings, but clearly here is an area in which further research is needed.

The practices and procedures contained in this book relate the results of a primary physician and psychologist collaborating to provide comprehensive health services to general medical patients. Eysenck has demonstrated in a series of studies in England that individuals with certain psychometric characteristics tend to have lower thresholds for stimulation, and lower pain thresholds, and to react differently to drug regimes.[4] The incorporation of psychological test results into the general medical protocols of patients would appear to be a fruitful area for exploration in this country.

As for combining full range psychological services—both psychodiagnostics and counseling/therapy—into ongoing general medical paractice, reports in the literature are meager. Follette and Cummings, in an investigation of psychological services within a prepaid health plan, drew the following conclusions:[5]

> patients suffering emotional distress were significantly higher users of both inpatient and outpatient medical facilities when compared to the average medical utilization rates;

> for those emotionally distressed patients receiving psychotherapy, a significant decrease in total medical utilization was observed when compared to a matched group of emotionally distressed patients not receiving psychotherapy;

> the declines noted in total medical utilization remained constant during five years following termination of psychotherapy;

> the most significant declines in total medical utilization occurred in the second year after the initial psychological interview, and those receiving only one psychotherapeutic session or brief psychotherapy (two to eight sessions) did not require additional psychotherapy to maintain lower medical utilization rates for the five-year period.

> patients seen for two or more years in regular psychotherapy demonstrated no overall decline in total outpatient utilization, since psychotherapy visits tended to supplant medical visits.

Such results confirm the observations and experiences reported in this book; namely, that pain and discomfort can be emotional, physical, or a combination of both, and if the emotional aspects are not recognized and dealt with, then overutilization of medical treatment occurs.

The efficacy of brief psychotherapy/counseling in the reduction of overutilization of medical services over a five-year period is even more significant in its cost effective implications. Many fears have been expressed by third party health providers that if psychotherapy/counseling is included as a part of comprehensive health care, then costs of health care would skyrocket. Certainly more research is needed; however, such fears appear unfounded.

Some primary physicians and psychologists may have doubts as to the effectiveness of spending an hour with a general medical patient attempting to provide rational education as to how emotions and physiological functioning interact. To the average man on the street, his autonomic nervous system is still somewhat of a mystery. The time spent in discussing with the patient how emotions, distress, worry, self-doubt, and anger can alter his physical state, or his cardiovascular or alimentary systems, is an effective approach to preventive medicine and for the nurturance of health, even on a "one-shot" basis. Whether such counseling is done by the physician or psychologist is immaterial. What *is* important is that such counseling is based upon valid physical and psychological findings.

Another concern, which might be hampering the collaborative efforts of primary physicians and psychologists in attempting to render broader total health care, is the doubt that general medical patients will accept combined medical-psychological services. First and foremost, psychological services including psychodiagnostic and psychosocial counseling, are not forced or fostered upon the general medical patient. Instead, as the primary physician and patient together formulate a health problem listing under POMIS, specific emotional/ behavioral health problems may evolve. As with any other type of health problem, a treatment plan is formulated. If the patient expresses a desire to ameliorate his identified emotional/behavioral health problems, then psychodiagnosis and psychosocial counseling are initiated. In such patients, who in effect have (1) been screened by self-realization of their emotional/behavioral distress and (2) indicate a willingness to seek amelioration or relief for such problems, their acceptance of the psychologist in the general medical setting is no different from their acceptance of the primary physician. Both are perceived as doctors concerned with the patient's pain or discomfort who are attempting to work with the patient as a partner in assessing the sources, alternatives, and possible solutions to restoring the patient to a state of health.

Future Areas for Collaboration between the Primary Physician and Psychologist

In this volume, primary physician–psychologist collaboration in the provision of health care services has been emphasized. Many other areas of mutual concern exist within the area of health research.[6]

1.   Much more needs to be done in the study of personality variables and the cause-and-effect relationship between incidence of specific diseases, the progress and course of the specific disease, and the reactions of the patient

to various treatment regimes. A long list of specific health conditions and diseases could be developed in which there appear to be psychologically related factors.

2. Why do patients not follow the medical advice of their physician about their state of health and its maintenance? What are the psychological determinants of such patient behaviors as brushing one's teeth or refraining from smoking, or taking one's prescribed medicine at the scheduled times? Such "simple" questions in today's modern medicine era may appear ridiculous, but the solutions to such questions are critical in total health care.

3. The assessment of individual patients' lifestyles as they relate to existing and near future illnesses, and the testing of primary physician intervention into the destructive aspects of such lifestyles, appear as rich areas for joint physician-psychologist collaboration.

4. How and why do individuals vary in their reactions to sickness, to recuperation, to recovery? What are the psychological attributes of certain individual patients who collapse under a minor health problem, while other patients cope with almost impossible life stress? (Current research efforts in coping with pending death typifies concerns within this area.)

5. What are the primary sources of persisting health care attitudes? What are the relationships between certain health attitudes and receptivity to preventive care activities?

6. How can psychological contributions of learning theory be better transposed to the rehabilitation of patients following disease or injury?

These and many other areas are of mutual concern to both physician and psychologist. For one or the other to attempt to answer such questions without the full collaboration of both disciplines appears ineffective in attempts to further comprehensive health. The author is convinced that joint collaboration of the two disciplines is a necessary trend of the future. Not only will the payoff be measured in cost effective terms by reducing utilization of limited medical resources, but it will also be demonstrated by the patient's obtaining a better understanding of his physical and psychological nature, which will aid him to better cope with the problems of living. This ultimate outcome is synonymous with medical and psychological definitions of health.

References

1. Kass, Leon R. The Pursuit of Health. *The Public Interest* 40(Summer 1975):29–30. Reprinted with permission of Leon R. Kass from *The Public Interest*, No. 40, Summer 1975. Copyright © 1975 by National Affairs, Inc.

2. Balint, M. *The Doctor, His Patient and the Illness*. New York: International Universities Press, 1957.

3. Ley, P. Comprehension, Memory and the Success of Communications with the Patient. *Journal of Institution Health Education* 10(1972):23-29.

4. Eysenck, H.J. *The Biological Basis of Personality*. Springfield, Ill.: Charles C. Thomas Press, 1967, pp. 34-74.

5. Follette, William T., and Cummings, Nicholas A. Psychiatric Services and Medical Utilization in a Prepaid Health Plan Setting. *Medical Care* 5(1967): 25-35.

6. APA Task Force on Health Research. Contributions of Psychology to Health Research. *American Psychologist* 31(1976):263-74.

About the Author

Allen Hodges has worked at community, state, and federal levels throughout his 28-year career, designing and rendering mental health/health services. He received the B.A. from the University of Minnesota, and the M.A. and Ph.D. from the University of Tennessee. Primary prevention in mental health, early diagnosis, interdisciplinary collaboration in service delivery, and mind-body interactions have been his long-standing professional concerns.

Based upon experiences with primary physician colleagues, Dr. Hodges is convinced that it is now time for a broader, more realistic, and comprehensive definition of health. Such a definition would create further impetus for collaboration between primary-care physicians and psychologists, and from his experiences and convictions came the motivation to write *Psychosocial Counseling in General Medical Practice.*